PENGUIN

SEVEN RULES TO RESET YOUR MIND
AND BODY FOR GREATER WELL-BEING

Dr Hansaji Yogendra is the director of The Yoga Institute, Mumbai, and president of the Indian Yoga Association (IYA). She is an exemplary yogi, philanthropist, scholar, internationally renowned spiritual guru, wellness mentor and thought leader. She is a global symbol of peace, balanced living and yoga. She is the leading face of the Householder Yoga and has personally conducted more than 1.5 lakh theoretical and practical yoga sessions.

Through the Householders Yoga Movement, it has been her mission to spread the teachings of Classical Yoga to the masses. She has trained over 1,00,000 yoga teachers who are dedicated towards creating awareness about yogic living in the world. She has enriched millions of lives with her wisdom by authoring and co-authoring more than 100 books. Dr Hansaji has a robust and compelling digital presence on various social media platforms and connects with millions worldwide. Under her guidance and training, millions have gained spiritual enlightenment, mastered mindfulness, unlocked hidden happiness and found balance in life.

Under her powerful leadership and guidance, The Yoga Institute has been awarded the Prime Minister's Award by honourable Prime Minister Narendra Modi for 'Outstanding Contribution in Yoga'. She brought about revolutionary changes in the institute by designing health systems, special techniques, health camp programmes and well-being modules that cater to a wide range of people across age, ethnicity and gender. She has led numerous research programmes in developing yogic solutions for common ailments.

Dr Hansaji is on the board of numerous national and international committees devising yoga syllabi and yoga policy. In a lifetime dedicated to service, she has been committed and devoted to helping others lead a healthy and happy life. With her humble nature, compassionate attitude and charming personality, Dr Hansaji continues to influence, shape and transform people's lives with her enlightening wisdom, and simple and effective methods.

7 RULES

TO RESET YOUR MIND AND BODY FOR GREATER WELL-BEING

Dr Hansaji Yogendra

**GLOBALLY ACCLAIMED
YOGA GURU, AUTHOR
AND SPIRITUAL LEADER
TO MILLIONS**

PENGUIN
ANANDA

An imprint of Penguin Random House

PENGUIN ANANDA

USA | Canada | UK | Ireland | Australia
New Zealand | India | South Africa | China

Penguin Ananda is part of the Penguin Random House group of companies
whose addresses can be found at global.penguinrandomhouse.com

Published by Penguin Random House India Pvt. Ltd
4th Floor, Capital Tower 1, MG Road,
Gurugram 122 002, Haryana, India

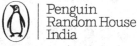

First published in Penguin Ananda by Penguin Random House India 2023

10 9 8 7 6 5 4 3 2 1

The contents of the book are general in nature and are only intended for
informational purposes. This book is not to be used as a substitute for
examination, diagnosis, treatment and advice by a trained, qualified and
recognized medical professional/healthcare provider, and readers are advised to
seek professional help while dealing with any medical, mental health, behavioural,
psychological and/or psychiatric issues, including but not limited to depression.
The author is not a qualified doctor nor claims to be in any manner whatsoever.

The views and opinions expressed in the book are those of the author and her
own understanding of materials referred to, and do not reflect or represent the
views and opinions of any other person. Neither the author nor the publisher shall
be liable for any loss, hurt or damage that may be caused due to the contents of
this book. while every effort has been made to report facts correctly in this book,
neither the author nor the publisher shall be liable for any errors, omissions or
inaccuracies that may be contained therein. Reader's discretion is advised.

The objective of this book is not to hurt any sentiments of, insult or cause offence
to any particular person, group or community, including those of any caste,
religious, regional, linguistic, gender or sexual identity.

ISBN 9780143456438

Typeset in Adobe Caslon Pro by Manipal Digital Systems, Manipal

www.penguin.co.in

Contents

Author's Note

The COVID-19 pandemic affected all of us in some way or the other. Some of us lost our jobs, others faced severe health challenges and some had to face the tragedy of losing someone they loved. The years of the pandemic were tough for all of us, to say the least. We all needed to reset our life from the issues that the pandemic exposed us to like financial insecurity, the importance of health and wellness, taking care of our mental health and giving time to our relationships. When Ms Vaishali Mathur of Penguin Random House India approached me to write a book, these were the thoughts that I was mulling over. I felt we needed a reset, not just because of the pandemic, but also because 'normal' life had more or less become a pattern rather than a journey of joy for most of us. I wanted to help people restructure their careers, social lives and emotions and also help them reset their relationship with food, exercise and sleep—the three foundational pillars of well-being.

I have written many books over the past decades on various aspects of yoga, well-being and consciousness. But for this book, I had something very special in mind—a practical and relatable formula for anyone who needed guidance on how to approach their life problems. The idea was to distil my years of knowledge in yoga, well-being and holistic living into something easy and simple that can be used by people in their daily lives. Don't be fooled by the words 'easy' and 'simple'. Easy and simple things are often the most powerful tools to help you change your life.

That was an ambitious goal which nevertheless got me quite excited about the book and I began to write. And as they say, anything creative first creates the creator and so it was with me as well. It was like I discovered something new within myself every time I sat down with my thoughts. But I finally identified seven different dimensions of modern life which were in dire need of a reset: perspective, emotions, social life, work-life, sleep, food and exercise. When these seven aspects are balanced, I don't see any impediment to you living a life of fulfilment and satisfaction. This does not mean that you won't face any challenges or obstacles in life. Rather, it means that when you learn from the 'reset formula' and apply it to your life, then you are well-equipped to face challenges with equanimity and confidence.

What sets this book apart for me is that it tries to meaningfully address and redress the issues in each of the seven categories and does not fixate on one or a few of them. These seven dimensions are, I believe, the bedrock of a healthy and abundant life. I have seen people, who are extremely successful professionally, neglect the other dimensions of their life and suffer for it. Either their personal relationships are in a state of irretrievable breakdown or the incessant demands of their professional lives have begun to take a toll on their body. Remember what you do to your body in your twenties and thirties, the body will do to you in your fifties and sixties. More often than not, this becomes a source of unhappiness and dissatisfaction in people's lives.

In my years at The Yoga Institute, I have observed that most of life's so-called problems begin to crop up when we tend to focus too much on one of these seven dimensions at the cost of others. Some people develop insomnia or issues related to stress when they devote too much time to their work or sacrifice their social life. Our body begins to suffer when we are imbalanced. It is so easy to ignore the needs of the body in the pursuit of all that we think is more important. But remember, nothing is more important than your health—emotional, physical and mental. The pandemic was a stern and grave reminder about this.

With this book, I wanted to reach out to all enterprising people and offer them The Yoga Institute's wisdom and legacy in the form of a modern, crisp and fun formula for success. I have always vouched that ambition or having goals is not bad, but focusing solely on them while ignoring everything else that is worthwhile is problematic. We are not defined by one thing, however important that one thing may seem to you at that particular moment in life. This idea has always been at the core of The Yoga Institute. Remember, you don't want to get to the top to realize that it's very lonely at the top. Your journey will be so much richer if your success entails a rich trove of relationships, experiences and memories.

So, what is the most important message of *Seven Rules to Reset Your Mind and Body for Greater Well-Being*? It's that you can have it all and the book's success formula is going to help you get there. Love what you do with every pore of your body but also live with every pore of your body. This book was written to help you wake up eager for the day's adventures, every single day.

With this book, I hope my voice helps you find your own so you can rediscover and reset your life!

Enjoy!

ONE

———

Reset Your Work Culture

'Don't get so busy making a living that you forget to make a life.'

—Dolly Parton

We were on our way to Mr Nirmal Bhatt's home for their annual Ganesh Chaturthi puja. As Anand, our driver, drove through the throngs of people celebrating Ganesh Visarjan, I couldn't help but think, *wouldn't it be nice to approach life as a carnival?* Then we could fill our lives with colours, music, dance, fun and purpose!

What do the world's best carnivals like Rio Carnival in Brazil, the carnival of Viareggio in Italy or the Mardi Gras in the USA have in common? They remind us how to celebrate life. They remind us how life is simple and that there is no need to become serious about it. We often put ourselves on the racetrack of life and keep running only to realize that there is never a finish line in the race to materialistic success. Yet we become so occupied with the race that we are only focused on what lies ahead, forgetting to pause and look at the beauty around us.

I asked Anand to be careful while driving through the dancing crowds. It was the fifth day of Ganesh Chaturthi and people were already beginning to come on the roads for the Visarjan processions. I knew it was not going to be an easy drive. Ganesh Chaturthi—you may call it a festival or a carnival—makes Mumbai come alive in a way like nothing else! I would say this is the world's largest carnival-like celebration, rejuvenating the busy city.

'Maa, it seems we are out today at the wrong time,' said a worried Anand while carefully navigating through each of the Ganapathi groups dancing to the deafening *dhols* on their way to Juhu beach.

'It is just this one lane; we will be through easily after we turn left. This is the main way to the beach,' I said, trying to calm his mind. Patience is the key to navigating not just traffic jams but also life problems. Sometimes we don't realize that a struggle is just a temporary phase, just one single lane. During such times, one usually either becomes restless or gives up.

'Anand, can you please switch on the GPS and check the fastest route?' asked Rohita softly, while trying to open the map app on her phone. The screen was refusing to load.

'Yes Rohita ji, sure', said Anand without taking his eyes off the road.

Rohita is a vibrant twenty-six-year-old woman who hails from Gujarat. She had visited our centre, The Yoga Institute, to do a teacher's training program. A brilliant and disciplined woman, she excelled in all the subjects of the course. She has, however, had her share of relationship problems—a breakup that had completely shattered her.

Work pressure and relationships are two major stressors prevalent among the youth today, who usually seem lost when it comes to handling them since they succumb very easily. Young people need guidance on how to handle these stressors. Rohita came to the institute to find herself again and is much stronger and braver now. After her course, she expressed her desire to continue being associated with the institute and aid us in serving people. I felt she could manage my schedule or assist me in my travels and welcomed her to the team.

'Rohita ji, I think we must take the second left; the GPS indicates that the first left is clogged with traffic,' said Anand.

'That's great, let's take that route,' said Rohita, relieved. 'Maa, wouldn't it be great if we had GPS for life which could warn us about our forthcoming problems, troubles and obstacles?'

Rohita's question was profound. With the help of technology, we have mastered the art of accurately predicting many future events, such as the movements of objects in outer space, the arrival of a storm or where a star would be positioned 100 years from today. We can even estimate when the universe will come to an end. But can we ever know what will happen to our life in the next moment?

'Well, that's an interesting thought,' I replied. 'We already have one. Your body is the best GPS you have. Every cell in your body is a sensor. All you have to do is listen to it. If your gut feeling tells you that something is wrong, listen to it. If your body tells you that it's stressed, then listen to it and take a step back. You just need to be mindful enough to sense them.' I reached for the water bottle and had a few sips of water. We passed the first left. Rohita thanked the app.

'Your mind can also become an indicator of things to come,' I continued. 'You just need to be in the present and a little clever. When you train your mind to see the cause behind every change that happens and the effect of every action, you slowly gain the intuition to see what might happen next.'

The mind is a mysterious element. It is a storehouse of all possibilities. Psychology of yoga helps one tap their stored potentials. I generally avoid discussing things that are supernatural and miraculous in nature, but sometimes we have to make people realize the hidden strength that lies within. Only when you realize you can, you will!

'Maa, is it possible for someone like me to become like that? Is it an easy process?' Rohita asked inquisitively.

I smiled at her and said, 'Yes, you can! Why not? Nothing is difficult if one is sincere, disciplined and focused on their goals. There are just three simple acts required to attain any goal: strong will, continued perseverance and letting go of all that doesn't contribute to your goal. Don't you think it is doable? Life goals are just that simple.' As the car took a left turn, I glanced over at Rohita who was still pondering over what had just been said.

'Hansama, everything sounds simple when you say it. Hopefully, I get to learn more and more from you, my life will be set then,' said Rohita, happily.

'Maa, we are almost there. We are reaching in a few seconds,' said Anand, softly.

'Finally!' exclaimed Rohita. She started folding her papers to put them inside her handbag. Her phone pinged with a notification: 'You have reached your destination.'

Sometimes I feel apps know you and your destiny more than anyone else in this world.

We had finally reached Mr Nirmal Bhatt's apartment in Lokhandwala, Andheri. The building was fifteen floors tall and decorated with glittering lights for the occasion of Ganesh Chaturthi. Nirmal and his wife Geeta, who had visited us last week, had invited us for a Ganesh Puja at their home. The couple have been associated with us for the last fifteen years.

Almost everyone who does a course with us expresses their wish to volunteer at the institute to help us in our mission to spread goodness and wellness. As I mentioned earlier to Rohita, to achieve any goals and objectives in life, one just needs three qualities:

1) Strong will
2) Continued perseverance
3) Letting go of all that doesn't contribute to your goals

But the most difficult thing is to maintain a strong will. I believe the trick to maintaining it is being in constant touch with like-minded people and communities that deal with topics of your interest. Mr Bhatt and Geeta did the same. Their strong will to progress physically and mentally did not falter because they were in constant touch with The Yoga Institute.

'Namaste Hansaji, thank you so much for coming,' said Mr Bhatt, walking towards us to receive us with Geeta, a few paces behind.

'How could I not come, Mr Bhatt? It is an important event,' I said, returning his greeting. 'Geeta, how are you? You look so fresh!'

'Yes ma'am, it is all due to Ganesh ji's *ashirvaad*,' she replied shyly.

'Let's move ahead, Hansaji,' said Mr Bhatt, pointing towards the elevator.

'Sure,' I replied.

We reached his flat on the thirteenth floor. The elevator was quicker than I expected.

As I entered their house, I could see almost a dozen people in the room, some of whom were familiar faces from the institute. They all walked towards me to greet me.

'Namaste Hansama, we are blessed to see you today,' said a young man with a big smile on his face.

'I am glad to be here and see you all too,' I replied.

'*Haan*, seeking your blessings, Maa', said the man with his hands still folded in namaste.

Sometimes, I think I am indebted to people for the love they show me. When you give love, you receive love. You will only receive what you give. Karma is so powerful.

Mr Bhatt interrupted us. 'Maa, please sit here,' he said, pointing to a seat next to him. I did so and noticed a Ganesh idol and the beautiful decorations around it.

The decoration around the Ganesh idol was a colourful array of flowers at the back with twinkling lights spiralling around the flowers. It was simple and minimalistic. I like elegant presentations. Simplicity has a unique beauty and power.

'Maa, please have juice,' Geeta said, holding a plate with different coloured juices. I prefer to eat and drink on standard time. Hence, I gently asked for just water. I took a few gulps.

A few people had gathered around and were expressing their views on my recent videos on YouTube. They wanted me to speak about certain topics on YouTube which they would like to hear. I made a mental note of them. One of the main principles of my life is listening to and fulfilling people's needs. I see it as my primary objective in life. Life is all about giving and not taking.

My principle in life has always been to focus less on what you want and more on what others want.

By doing this:

- You become clever at understanding people around you.
- You have lesser expectations.
- You know how to make people happy.

All three are the roots of any successful relationship, either in personal or professional life.

'Maa, please we would like you to start the *aarthi*,' said Mr Bhatt.

'Yes, sure!' I said and walked towards the Ganesh idol.

'Where is your son Aarav? I don't see him anywhere,' I asked.

'He is working from home nowadays; he is in his bedroom. He is working on some urgent project,' said Bhatt.

I could sense some discomfort in his reply. Something was surely wrong.

'Maa, please,' Bhatt handed the aarthi plate to me with lit camphor.

As I did the aarthi, the energy of the room changed. Everyone started singing and clapping in harmony. This is what festivals do to people. They brighten the day. Festivals connect us to the beauties of life and remind us to acknowledge its beautiful colours.

'Bhatt, you do the aarthi now,' I said, handing the plate over after a minute.

'Thank you, Maa,' said Bhatt.

'Maa, please sit,' Geeta insisted after seeing me standing for a long while.

Geeta sat down next to me. I could sense she wanted to say something so I broke the silence to make her feel at ease.

'How is Aarav doing?' I asked casually.

'Maa, he is . . .' She paused for a moment and continued. 'Last month, he experienced severe chest pain. We had to take him to the hospital immediately. Doctors said he had a minor heart attack.'

I was a little shocked hearing this. 'What is his age?' I asked

'He will be turning twenty-nine next month,' she said. Her voice was shaky.

The average age for the onset of cardiac diseases has been decreasing constantly. According to the Indian Heart Association, almost 25 per cent of cardiac arrests in men in India were noticed below the age of forty.

Above all, our sedentary lifestyles have contributed to the rising incidence of cancer too.

Let me tell you, no illness occurs naturally. There is always a cause and I believe it is always psychological, your own mental state. The present work culture is playing a major role in burnout in today's youth. We are the cause of our problems. Humanity is going wrong somewhere as a whole.

'You should have told me immediately when it happened last month,' I said. 'How is his condition now? Is he better?'

'He is taking medications. I wanted him to visit the institute to help treat this condition. But Maa, he doesn't believe in yoga. He still thinks that things can get better with just medicine.'

This is one of the major misunderstandings people across the globe have, that medicine alone can solve all the problems. But in fact, the cause of the problems remains unaddressed. According to my experience, a majority of diseases are due to faulty attitudes and are psychosomatic. Our perceptions and patterns of thinking are the cause of every change that happens in our bodies. Our mind is the cause of our state of the body.

'Maa, I want you to talk to him,' she said hopefully. 'After all that happened last month, he hasn't learned. He is still busy with his work and has no time for even a short festive celebration!'

'I will talk to him. Do not worry,' I assured her.

She thanked me and immediately went to the other room, where I guessed Aarav was working. In the meantime, I could see Bhatt offering the *prasad* to everyone. Geeta came out smiling, Aarav following her with a blank face.

I could see strong dark circles around his eyes. He looked overweight and his skin was a little dry.

He needs sleep and hydration, I thought.

Sleep and hydration are two things today's young workforce neglects.

'Namaste Hansama, I am sorry to have missed the aarthi. I was on a conference call with my team,' Aarav spoke with an evidently forced smile.

'Aarav, don't be sorry. It is totally fine. I am happy to see you,' I said, trying to make him feel better.

Geeta came near and whispered, 'Maa, if you don't mind, can I arrange for you to go to the next room?'

'Yes sure, great!' I agreed.

The Conversation That Mattered the Most

While moving into the room, I asked Aarav, 'Beta, when are you planning to get married?'

'I need some more time, Maa,' he said a little shyly. 'I don't feel settled. I need to settle first.'

'So what are you doing about it, Aarav?' I asked.

'Maa, currently I am occupied with multiple things. I'm trying to get a flat for myself. This house would not be comfortable to stay in after my marriage. I am looking to buy a three-bedroom house in this neighbourhood. I'm trying for a house loan and doing my best to gather the base money within a year or two. Only then can I think about marriage.'

'But this is a two-bedroom house, right? Wouldn't that be enough for you, your spouse and your parents?' I asked casually.

'I feel it would be a bit too crowded,' he said seriously.

I understood then that he had set himself some big dreams and goals.

'How is your health now, Aarav? I got to know about your attack a few minutes back.'

'I am totally fine. It was just a little pain. You know how my mom is about such things, she just worries unnecessarily. I'm taking my medicines and I am totally fine.'

'Aarav, she is worried because she loves you,' I replied softly.

Sometimes, we fail to understand the reasons of the people who love us the most or we take them for granted.

I continued, 'It could be a little painful. But don't take it lightly. These are symptoms of what harm could happen in the future. You should respect your body, respect yourself and not neglect your health. Just be a little mindful, Aarav.'

'Maa, I'm fine. It was just that I have been a little occupied during the last few months,' said Aarav, as if nothing serious had happened.'

'Let me tell you about a case . . .'

I started to explain to him an incident that had happened five years ago. 'There was a brilliant student in our ashram, in his late twenties. His name was Satyam. He had big dreams and he certainly could have made them come true. After his course at the institute ended, he told me he had come up with a big idea for a business. He estimated that the demand for his product would be immense. He was going to get started with it soon and I wished him the very best. A couple of years later, I heard that he had been nominated for an emerging entrepreneur award. I was not surprised; the boy had great instincts. But a few months later, I heard of his demise. He'd died of a heart attack. I was shocked! A young man in his twenties getting a heart attack! Turns out he had been working for twenty hours a day and his routine was all over the place. He had stopped listening to his body and had kept pushing himself. He had certainly achieved worldly success but at the cost of leaving the world.'

Do Not Work in a Hurry

This reminded me of an interesting experiment done by Darley and Batson in 1973. They recreated the parable of the Good Samaritan from the Bible.

'Let's examine another instance of haste,' I said, settling into the sofa. 'In 1973, these two researchers conducted an interesting experiment. They shortlisted a few students for observation and divided them into three categories. The students were not told that they were part of an observational experiment. The first group of students was summoned on a high emergency basis to reach a building within 2 minutes. While on their way to the hall, they had placed an injured man who was unable to get up. The study was to observe how many of the students will help him. Similarly, the second category of students was summoned on a moderate emergency basis and was supposed to reach the building in say 5 minutes. The third category was not given any specific time to adhere to when summoned. Tell me, which category would have had the most helpers?' I asked Aarav.

'Wouldn't it depend on a person's character? Anyone having basic humanity would help the injured.' he answered.

'You are right, the compassionate ones would help. But the results were obvious: "Overall 40 per cent offered some help to the victim. In low-hurry situations, 63 per cent helped, medium-hurry 45 per cent and high-hurry 10 per cent." Do you feel that students from the first category were less compassionate?' I asked again.

'I'm sure they were nice people, it's just that they were rushed and couldn't attend to the needy.'

'Yes Aarav, exactly. The same happens to us. When the body needs attention and we fail to give it that attention because we are in a hurry we end up ignoring the damage it's undergoing.'

At this point, his phone beeped. He took his phone out and his expression said that he wanted to look at it. Then he hesitated and put it back in.

I asked him, 'Has it ever happened that you are frantically looking for your phone everywhere, but it turns out that it was in your pocket the whole time?'

Aarav grinned, 'Well, yes. Many times, in fact!'

'That is what happens when our mind is in a rush. It makes us absent-minded. When you hurry thoughtlessly, you miss what you already have with you. We forget the basics of living in the pursuit of quick success. Satyam had everything in life: talent, skills, money, success, etc. But then he lost the most precious thing: his life. What value does anything hold if it is going to cost you your life? Respect life by respecting your body. Do not be in a hurry. Learn to relax!'

I was telling him this story not to alarm him but to make him realize the right thing. In today's world, people desire rapid promotions in their careers and are ready to give up anything for it, including their health, family life and peace of mind. Let me tell you—promotion is not equal to progress. Progress should always be across all dimensions of life, not just the professional. People fail to recognize that they have personal, social and family lives. Society has conditioned us to believe that career or financial progress means complete success.

'Now tell me Aarav, do you think Satyam was doing the right thing?'

I could see Aarav thinking deeply. His expression was a mix of agreement and disagreement.

'He should have taken care of himself, Maa. But how can we give up on our goals? If someone needs basic comforts and security, there isn't much choice. I want to buy a three-BHK home and I have to buy it before I am married. It is a need for which I must work hard.'

Simplicity Is the Key to Reducing Work Stress

I explained to him, 'Look, goals are always going to be a part of our lives. They should be! It's good to dream big. What's not good is always being in a hurry and neglecting other aspects of life which are equally important. If you strike a balance, you can go about things the right way. You already have your present home, which you must learn to appreciate and accept. Be content with it till you achieve what you want ahead. Remember, you create your own needs. Some needs didn't come to you but you created them. You created the need for a 3BHK. And your needs are perfectly fine; just make sure that they do not harm your personal health and family's well-being.'

Aarav was nodding in agreement.

'We are also prone to create more needs than necessary. Our entire lifestyle is highly influenced by such attitudes. You must learn to recognize which needs are important and which are not.'

At this moment, the door opened halfway, and Geeta peeked around it.

'Maa, would you like to eat now?' she asked.

'No dear, thanks,' I said politely.

'Please let us know if anything is required,' she offered.

'Sure,' I waved and smiled.

As she closed the door, I recalled an observation my husband Dr Jayadev had once shared with me. He had been the epitome of right living.

Do Not Fill Your Plate

'Aarav, notice this the next time you attend a wedding dinner. There, you will find three kinds of people. First, there are those who pile their plates with everything available on the counter. Second, there are those who are tempted to add something to their plate after noticing the food on other peoples' plates even though they know they won't be able to finish it and third, there are those who only take a limited amount of food based on how much they are certain they can finish and they add food to their plate gradually only when they need to. The third kind of people are mindful; they don't pile food on their plates beyond what they can easily consume. The behaviour such people show around the dinner table reflect their fundamental attitudes towards life as well. Some individuals are like the first kind—adding more and more needs to their lives to the point of breaking. Some are like the second kind—motivated to add extra needs to their lives after comparing their situation with others. And finally, the third one, whom we all should be like—add to your plate only when required. **Learn to be like that; don't overburden yourself with unnecessary**

work pressure. Instead, concentrate on how much you can accomplish using a calm state of mind.

'We need to accept the fact that sometimes our lifestyle itself is what financially drains us. Now let me ask you a simple question. Who decorated the Ganapathi *mandap*?'

Aarav quickly responded, 'Mom and Dad. They did so in a single evening.'

I nodded. 'What I liked the most about the decoration is the simplicity with which it has been done. It is elegant, beautiful and impressive. The objective is still met within the simplicity. In life too, one of the easiest solutions for the most complex challenges is the philosophy of simple living. I don't mean to say that you must live the life of a sanyasi in just a few clothes. What I mean is: spend your money mindfully. Do not create unnecessary needs. Simpler living means minimizing your requirements. We have all experienced the need to live simply at some point in our life. I am reminded of the initial three months of the first COVID-19 lockdown.'

Aarav was just listening keenly with a face that expressed deep thinking and introspection.

'When the lockdown happened, some of our residential students could not go back to their countries. They stayed at our campus for almost a year. Some were from Russia, Italy, Estonia, Brazil, the USA and some were Indians from other states. In one way, they felt fortunate to have gotten the opportunity to spend more time at the institute. The institute was completely sealed for a year and no insider was allowed to go out. One rainy morning, I had just entered the hall for a short session with our residential students. I said namaste and sat on the dais. Although the place was secure, social distancing was being practised even during the classes with students seated more than a metre apart. I asked them to tell me one thing that they had learned during the lockdown. I wanted to know their observations. Many interesting answers were offered: "Nature is unimaginably more powerful than us humans," said a Brazilian *sadhika*. "Life can turn around in no time. Uncertainty is the only reality of it," said another student. "Many human beings helped each other, irrespective of nationality, colour, creed, religion and caste. The lockdown united us," answered an Indian. Other students offered equally fascinating perspectives on what they'd learned and I was impressed.'

'Then came the most interesting answer. A Russian student said, "Hansama, I think I have learned to live my life with minimum things. I realized things are still the same without the shopping, restaurant outings, travelling, etc. Life is more peaceful with our needs kept at a minimum." What this girl said is 100 per cent true. We all have experienced this minimalistic living.

'How many clothes have you purchased during the lockdown? How much did you spend on travelling? How much did you spend on restaurant food? Just make a rough estimate. It would be almost negligible. How much money would you have saved by not indulging in mindless shopping and eating?'

Our conversation was again interrupted by a series of notification beep sounds. Aarav looked at the phone for a second and then kept the phone away. He ignored the notifications.

I continued, 'A major work-related stressor is always a race of earning more and achieving financial security. We put ourselves under tremendous pressure by following a lifestyle that is filled with too many needs. Simple living, on the other hand, makes you content with what you have and saves a lot of your income. For instance, a man who earns Rs 50,000 may be unhappy and consider it insufficient. He may want a lakh per month instead. The person feels the same after reaching 1 lakh after a few years. This is because he has changed his needs according to the higher income, such that at every point of his life, he is unsatisfied with present outcomes.

'Learning to live simply can reduce peoples' stress considerably. Let me give you a simple reminder formula to follow before you even spend a rupee. Keep three things in mind before making a purchase:

1) Is it an essential need?
2) If it is a need, ask yourself is it affordable?
3) If it is affordable, then try to find the best products available around the same price.

'This mental exercise may sound very simple, but it does help prevent you from buying or doing something mindlessly. This should be practised for every rupee you spend. Aarav, you can have sufficient savings with your present income. Just be clever in your expenditures. As I said earlier, you create your needs. These needs are sometimes created by looking at others. We constantly compare our attainments and success with those of others. If that is the case, you would never be satisfied with the results.'

Comparison

I leaned back. 'Tell me, what makes a peacock beautiful and what makes a swan beautiful?'

Aarav thought about it for a couple of seconds. 'I think both are beautiful'

'How come?' I questioned. 'The former has beautifully colourful feathers; the latter is almost pure white. How can both be beautiful?'

'The swan's beauty lies in the simplicity of its pure whiteness.' said Aarav. 'The peacock's beauty lies in the complexity of its colourful feathers. Both are unique in their own ways.'

'Exactly Aarav, it would be foolish to compare both. Both have their own character and beauty. The swan is beautiful in its simplicity. You too can train yourself to live a simple life. It has its own beauty. I see peace in it. But then we compare our journey with others and put ourselves under unnecessary peer pressure. Everyone is on their separate journey; one must learn to accept and enjoy it.'

Aarav spoke, 'I agree that such comparisons put us under unnecessary pressure and that sometimes we don't even realize we are developing more needs based on comparison. But it is difficult to control our temptations for luxuries and hold ourselves back from competing in this world. It's difficult to hold myself back when everyone around me is progressing quickly.'

'When someone is growing quickly, they would have their share of personal problems which the world might never come to know of. Are any of your guests today aware that you have a heart issue?' I wanted to bring him to a point of realization.

'No, only you know,' he muttered.

'To the world, you are a successful man, but hardly anyone knows about your family or personal health. This is the illusion in which we live today. People may appear successful and happy on the outside, but may not be so internally. You must grow at the right pace. The journey must be smooth. You must compete with yourself and not others.'

'Sorry, Maa, I didn't understand the "competing with self" part,' he said inquisitively.

'What I mean is that in today's time, you must work more on upgrading your skills. Do you know the progress the world underwent in the last thirty years has happened within the last three years? We are growing quickly. The market changes quickly; businesses and professions become outdated in no time. Upgrading yourself to keep up is necessary to avoid unnecessary trouble in the future.'

I could see he was glued to the conversation, his eyes unblinking. But the focus and concentration were shattered by and the loud sound of dhol playing down in the street, indicating that some Ganesh Visarjan procession may be on the way. Suddenly there was a silence between us while waiting for the loud music to fade away. He was thinking deeply which was evident from his legs. He was shaking them subconsciously.

'Maa, what should I do now?' he asked, genuinely concerned.

I decided that a story might help. 'An organization held a one-of-a-kind cooking competition. Participants in this contest were given the option of describing the dish of their dreams—something they'd love to have but had never eaten. Some participants said they would love to eat the royal dishes that the kings used to eat, while others named specific cuisines from all over the world.

'Top chefs were called to cook the amazing dishes. They could prepare any cuisine from around the world. After everyone had submitted their preferences, the chefs got ready to cook. After a while, the contest began. The participants were given only 5 minutes to finish the entire dish. The winner was to be the person who finished their plate in less than that time.

'When the buzzer rang,' I continued, 'everyone began eating as quickly as they could. The buzzer rang again in 5 minutes to signal the end of the time limit. Just when all those who finished the dish got excited about winning a big prize the host revealed a twist in the competition: he asked those who had finished their meal within 5 minutes to name the ingredients that were used to make their dream dish. Participants were confused since no one had paid attention to the ingredients; their minds had concentrated on the clock and they had simply eaten to win the competition.

'This is exactly how we live our lives. We are provided a variety of wonderful things, but we are often in such a rush that we neglect them and completely focusing on something takes away our peace of mind. Just like the participants who never got to enjoy the delicious dishes that were made with a variety of exquisite ingredients.

'So, to answer your question, we need variety as part of our living and that too in balance. This is the key to not only your health but also to your professional success. If you fill your life with just one kind of activity, then your mind is going to react to it with stress and depression. In the pursuit of money and success, we often forget the other essential aspects of living and underestimate such activities. But these activities play a significant role in our physical, mental and emotional health. All you need to do is bring balance and variety to your work culture. Break the monotony of work!

'Reset your work culture by following these four fundamental tips:

- Be health-centred in work
- Engage in recreational activities
- Invest in yourself
- Be creative in your profession

'All of these must become part of your work-life. Such a balance would only enhance your productivity in your profession. We fail to understand the power of small things in life.'

Be Health-Centred in Work

'Aarav, how long do you sit while working?' I asked.

'Hmm, I can't say for sure. I have never observed,' he said politely.

'Fine, how often do you walk while working?'

'I get up mostly for bathroom or food breaks,' he said, confidently.

'I can assume you might be sitting for three or four hours at a stretch. That is where we make mistakes—we forget about our body and its health while working intensely. You know these simple acts are the causes of weight gain, bad posture, orthopaedic ailments and back problems, etc., in today's youths,' I explained.

One of the major causes of health problems is the changing work culture in the last two decades. The nature of work now is such that there are fewer physical movements throughout the day. And this affects the metabolism severely. Your body tends to stay in resting metabolism for a longer part of the day and this, in turn, leads to the accumulation of fats in the body. Also sitting in an incorrect posture for a long period does lead to various orthopaedic issues. The tragedy is that many are unaware of the cause of the problems. All it takes are some simple yet mindful actions to correct the mistakes that we make while working to prevent the development of any serious ailments.

'Aarav, you are making a mistake here,' I cautioned. 'Get up every half hour and go for a short 2-minute walk inside your office or outside. Or you can climb up and down the stairs for a couple of minutes. This sounds simple. You might even doubt how big a change it can bring. But believe me, it could just prevent the development of all the problems that would arise due to your sedentary lifestyle. Also, how long have you been having those dark circles around your eyes?'

'They started appearing three years ago back, Maa. They continue to become darker. I tried some facials to lighten them but they keep reappearing,' he answered.

'This is again due to sitting for hours in front of the desktop and watching the screen without blinking. Here, try the 20-20 rule, for every 20 minutes, close your eyes for 20 seconds. This will do wonders for your eyes. You don't need facial, you just need to practice clever management of yourself during work hours. Learn to be observant of your body and mind during that time.

'I also just remembered your absence during aarthi. Why didn't you come?' I asked

'Maa, I had mentioned this to you earlier—I had been on a conference call,' he said.

'Yes, this is where we make mistakes. It was just a matter of 15 minutes. You could have shifted the call by 15 minutes or maybe 30 minutes. Did you have that choice?'

'Yes, it could have been possible.'

'Prioritize other activities too. The pooja event is the kind of break you need to keep giving yourself during the day,' I said.

Engage in Recreational Activities

It is important to engage in activities that rejuvenate you. In the race for promotions and quick monetary gains, we often forget another important aspect of our life: entertainment. We don't even realize how certain fun activities just gradually disappear from our lives as we age. I would like to mention here that children's games are the world's best stress busters. As we grow older, we forget to play indoors and outdoors, we forget to trek and we forget our hobbies. It is time to bring such activities back into our lives. If you can't do so daily, at least take time to engage yourself in some recreational activity during the weekend.

Indian festivals have their purpose rooted in this cause. They act as breaks from usual life activities and teach us to celebrate the ethics and beauty of life. The advantage of having so many festivals is that they break the monotony of routine.

'Aarav, recreation should become an essential part of your routine. Pick up the activity you love the most. It could be art, sports, travelling or anything else you like. Just bring it into your life. For instance, what do you love doing the most other than your IT work?'

Aarav replied immediately, 'I love bird watching, but I used to do that long back. I even hold a university certificate for this.'

'Wah! That's nice. Why don't you just start doing it either in the evenings or on weekends? You must add recreational activity into your life again. You need happy and pleasant hormones,' I said. I could see a lot of ease in his face by now. There was no deep thinking or confusion in his expressions, it was just pure agreement and acceptance.

We are, in one way, a bundle of chemicals. **Life is mysterious and it holds infinite potential. The aspect of life that can tap into this potential is spirituality.** People have got different notions about spirituality. However, I am referring only to self-development at physical, mental, emotional and intellectual levels. One must put more effort into understanding the larger aspects of life, body and mind.

Invest in Yourself

'Aarav, thirdly you must invest time in self-development. I am not speaking of developing skills related to your profession. I'm referring to the practice of increasing your understanding of life, your mind and the universe. Get in touch with your roots. You can do it in many ways, for example, read books that would make you more mature and wiser; books that teach you how to live life. I always say the best time to read such books is in bed, half an hour before sleep. They have the tremendous capacity of changing your subconscious thinking pattern. Or you can get in touch with some communities that work on health and wellness. The Yoga Institute is always open for you—stay in touch with our activities. Doing so shall infuse life with new meaning, allowing you to view the broader picture of it.'

'Maa, I have been thinking about this for the last couple of years to do some course from the institute but couldn't take time out. I see my parents going to institute and I have personally seen how drastically they have changed over the years. I want to come. Are there any weekend programs available?'

I could sense the excitement in his voice. 'Yes, sure. There are. You can come to our weekend programmes, or you can attend my Satsang every Sunday at 9.30 a.m.,' I said.

'Sure Maa, I will be there next Sunday,' he said with assurance.

I continued coming back to the topic at hand. 'Let's discuss one last thing: how to bring creativity to your work and avoid pressure.'

Be Creative in Your Work

'Remember, you are going to spend a major part of the day working. Make it exciting. Be creative in your methods,' I said. 'Do you remember what I said regarding the way you should approach your work?' I asked and I could immediately sense a discomfort on his face. It was almost like a direct test, as if he was being grilled in an interview.

'Never work in a hurry, work in a relaxed state . . .'

'Generate an attitude of simple living and do not spend money mindlessly. And Maa, you stressed on how important it is to keep updating ourselves in our profession and . . . yes that's all,' he finished, relieved.

'Good, but you forgot one important thing. Do not put yourself under pressure by comparing yourself with others. You are on your journey, while others are on theirs. That's all you need to know. I am saying this not just for your health but also for your progress in your professional space. Life is not one-dimensional—there are many sides and angles to it. Learn to live a balanced life. Reset the way you work.'

I would like to stop the story here. The conversation we had that evening left a strong mark on Aarav's mind. He made dramatic changes to the way he approaches work culture. He finally bought a house three years after our conversation. He is happily married and his chest pain never recurred. He expresses his gratitude every time he visits the institute.

Can you all be like Aarav? Ready to reset! He chooses to keep his phone notifications off and give his full attention to the person who is speaking. There is no escape from work, but we do have the choice to prioritize our work and maintain the right state of mind while at work. Do not run mindlessly which would drain your life's energy in the longer run. I like an analogy I read somewhere that was shared by an American politician. If a lion hunted and ate only field mice, it would probably starve slowly to death. This is because the energy spent hunting and eating is much more than the calories the field mice can provide. Much like us, we keep working mindlessly and it drains our energy in the longer run. Life is always mouldable. It only takes your choice to initiate it. Be the Aarav who put the phone away for the moment, for the sake of his health.

It is time to reset!

TWO

Reset Your Perception

'You see things not as they are but as you are.'
—Anthony de Mello

Water trickled listlessly from the hose in my hands as the evening sun splashed hues of emerald and gold around me.

'Jagtap, check the water-level in the tank,' I said and smiled at the ease with which our gardener scampered towards it. He seemed like the many squirrels that dart around our garden at The Yoga Institute. As if sensing my reference to squirrels, a particularly agile one sped past me, right up the leafy boughs of our kailashpati tree. A student-favourite, the kailashpati bloomed perennially, sharing its beauty and joy with us throughout the year. My eyes followed my furry friend up and up the old, gnarled tree and seeing it dash between the flowers joyfully, I gained an insight into why students loved the majestic tree. With its six reddish-pink petals encircling a hood-shaped tentacle, the kailashpati flower has an inexplicable magic; the same magic that's at the heart of creation. This, I have always known in my heart, is what makes the kailashpati take you on long introspective journeys; journeys that are infinitely soothing and rewarding.

The unique kailashpati has a spiritual significance across the globe. The petals of the kailashpati flower are believed to be the seat of Vishnu, resting on the primal serpent *Adisesha*. The hooded tentacle aspect of the flower represents Adisesha reposing over Vishnu. Others believe that Shiva resides in the hooded centre while Buddhists believe it is Buddha who meditates there. Many other stories surround this beautiful and fragrant flower. Sometimes students ask me, 'Whose belief is right? Who lives at the heart of the flower? Shiva, Buddha or Vishnu?' Try as I might, I can't suppress a smile at the human mind's need to have rigid boundaries and clear definitions instead of simply enjoying the kailashpati's beauty like the squirrel. But, in the rational, practical world that we call home, it's a justified question. So, I always respond with, 'To each their own,' often to the gentle annoyance of my students. Annoyed, perhaps, by my refusal to give them certainties in stories about cosmic flowers. But just as each petal of the kailashpati is unique, so is each story around it and so are the many opinions that surround us in life.

Look at things from all sides. Do we need answers or opinions to be right or another to be wrong? Or would it be better to look at how each petal goes into the making of a rare flower?

Things, situations, people; everything has multiple dimensions and is the better for it. You have within you the choice of seeing all sides or narrowing in on one. If we didn't allow differences of opinion, we would still have believed in the idea of a flat earth with the sun revolving around it. We must respect everyone's views, ideologies and ways of living.

Just then, Jagtap exclaimed from the ladder leading to the water tank, 'Maa, the tank is almost full; let me check the motor.' He climbed down quickly and rushed to the motor. I observed how nimbly he had scaled up and down the ladder. 'Practice,' I thought, 'makes a man not just perfect but also extraordinary!' Sometimes, certain things seem impossible or beyond us, but it's merely a matter of spending sufficient time to master them.

Things Become Simple or Complex Based on How You Deal with Them

I saw Jagtap oiling the motor and restarting it and soon, water gushed out of the pipe in my hands. I saw the sun gleam on every droplet on the leaves; it was incomparably beautiful. If we could just be open to the many wonders that surround us, life would be so full of simple joys, such as the scent of pepper mingling with the aroma of the damp earth.

'The black pepper has matured,' I said. 'We'll have to pluck it soon.'

'Yes Maa, I will,' Jagtap said with a toothy smile. Our gardeners all have the same expression of happiness every time a spice, herb or fruit matures. Their sense of achievement from having patiently nurtured life is reflected in these smiles as they see the literal fruit of their work.

Black pepper has an interesting history. Once known as black gold, pepper was extremely valuable than gold. The spice had originated in India, which was the only country to cultivate it back then. But as Portuguese ships landed on Indian shores and a lucrative spice trade began, demand sky-rocketed and the world valued it more than gold. But today, pepper has returned to its humbler roots. Don't you think the value of things change over time? That which was an invaluable asset today might become commonplace tomorrow or vice versa. Remember how valuable VCRs were once and how they are forgotten now? What makes something valuable? Is there some certainty in value? The easy answer is that value changes with time and perception. At a point, VCRs and pepper were considered invaluable but as time passed, people's perception of their worth changed.

> It is important at each point in life to identify what you should value the most and what you shouldn't.

I finished watering our plants and made my way out of the garden. As I neared the security cabin, I could hear someone arguing with our security guard. Coming closer, I noticed it was Mike, a residential student of ours from Spain, arguing with the guard. He was in his mid-thirties and had joined the Institute for a three-month teacher training program, which he was only two weeks into. He was red-faced and flustered; his shirt was wrinkled, his hair unkempt. He was holding a bulky bag in hand and seemed worried and distraught. As Mike saw me walking towards him, he lowered his voice and smiled, albeit uncomfortably. I smiled back.

'Namaste, Maa,' he greeted with folded hands.

'Namaste, Mike, how are you?' I asked.

'O-okay, Maa,' he mumbled, unsure of himself. I knew if this was okay, then nothing would ever be okay again.

'You don't look like you're okay. You seem worried. Is everything really fine?' I asked insistently.

Before Mike could reply, our guard interrupted us. 'Maa, he wants me to get his clothes delivered for laundry. I did this for him during the last couple of days even though it was not my job. I thought he was unwell, so I helped him. And he seems perfectly fine but now he wants me to do it every day.'

I looked at Mike, expecting his side of the story. He began, 'Maa, I have not stepped out of the campus for five days. I know it is my duty to do my personal chores like laundry. But I don't *want* to step outside the institute. I don't like the place outside and I just want to stay indoors.' He looked sulky, not unlike a small child who had made up his mind about something. I half-expected him to stomp his foot in anger.

'But why?' I asked. 'What's wrong outside?'

'Maa, that's a long story. I don't think you have the time,' he replied.

'Do not worry about my time. Come meet me in my sitting room in 10 minutes,' I told him.

I soothed the ruffled feathers of the guard and started walking towards the building. Opening the door, I saw Dr Jayadeva, my husband, seated in the living room, flipping through some pages; probably the 'Positive Points' assignment submitted by our seven-day health camp students. An important exercise of this popular camp that involves writing about ten positive things that happened in your day and submitting them to be reviewed the next morning. This simple exercise has the power to alter the way we think. It encourages you to be grateful, think positively and see the beauty in every person, event and activity.

Ten Positive Points a Day Keep Gloomy Thoughts Away

Try this simple yet profound exercise: every day before going to bed (or alternatively, early morning), recall the events of the previous twenty-four hours and note down at least ten positive events of the day. It could be anything—maybe you caught up with a friend after a long time, helped a stranger, saw something beautiful, or simply were happy during some parts of the day.

Write down ten positive things that you experienced during the day. This is a powerful, subconscious exercise that will strengthen your mind and make you notice the beauty around and within you, something which normally escapes our attention. Most of us usually tend to notice only the worst aspects of an event or situation. But this exercise trains the mind to see the brighter parts of it. Try this for a week! If you notice a considerable change in your mood, which you would, then continue it as a regular part of your routine.

Dr Jayadeva used to carefully peruse the positive events experienced by our students and track their progress. He would then suggest suitable practices to each of them to aid their journey within. I silently walked past him to the room where I occasionally met with students and teachers to listen to their queries or plan upcoming camps and courses. As I entered, I saw Mike settled on the couch. He smiled a bit sheepishly as I sat down facing him.

'So, Mike, what's bothering you?' I said encouragingly.

'Maa, I haven't been able to manage my personal work for a few days because I haven't stepped out of the institute. I've been unable to get my fruits, toiletries, laundry and, more importantly, I've been unable to get a haircut,' he said irritably, shaking his shoulder-length hair. I knew a lot more than a haircut was brewing inside his head.

'But who stopped you from going outside?' I asked.

'No one, Maa. I decided not to go out. I don't like anything outside!' Again, he looked like a little child, his face all red and flustered. 'The places, the people. Nothing! Nobody understands my language and I don't understand theirs. I had such a horrible experience five days ago! I have decided to stay indoors now. I just want to stay inside campus Maa. In fact, I might as well quit the course since it is becoming difficult to manage my personal chores. But I also do not want to miss the opportunity to learn from you and Dr Jayadeva or finish this wonderful course.' Mike almost exploded, sharing his conclusion vehemently, all the while looking rather miserable.

'But what horrible experience did you have?' I asked, curious but also a bit taken aback.

'Well, last Saturday, I went to Kala Ghoda to buy some handicrafts and kurtas. This was my first outing in Mumbai on my own and I was excited about the trip. I left the institute around 9.00 a.m. in the morning and walked towards the Santa Cruz railway station. But what a nasty surprise—the streets were outrageously filthy! The walls along it were piled high with waste and garbage and full of paan spittle. Rodents like rats and mice were roaming the streets with complete abandon, which were full of potholes, filled with muddy water from the previous day's rain—breeding grounds for the myriads of mosquitoes and flies that were buzzing about. I accidentally fell into one of those potholes and soaked myself in dirty water!' he recounted with horror.

Now I started to understand and reassuringly placed my hand on his shoulder, nodding encouragingly for him to go on. Mike looked at me, unsure about himself and pretty much everything, but continued.

'I reached the station somehow but boarding the train proved to be another nightmare,' he recounted. 'It was a mad rush. Each train that came in was already full of people, yet at the station, more people jostled, pulled and pushed to board the train. The train would start moving and yet, people kept trying to board. It was awful to think of what would have happened if someone slipped and fell onto the tracks!' Mike paused and closed his eyes, reliving the experience.

He gathered himself. 'I couldn't get onto any train for quite some time. Every time I tried, I would be pushed or elbowed away by the desperate crowd. Some even yelled at me for blocking their path. This happened five or six times,' he said with a small shudder.

His aversion to the world outside the campus was becoming clearer, but I sensed there was more to his story and encouraged him again to go on. After a pause, he continued retelling the experience that had left him so shaken, even days later.

'And while the railway station had been terrible, inside the train it was even worse! The compartments were so crowded, I could hardly breathe with someone's head or even armpit directly in my face. Yet at every stop, more and more people got in. For a few stations, I hung precariously from the door. I was frightened of being pushed out onto the rails under another speeding train! Gradually, however, I managed to inch further into the compartment but that wasn't much better as now people had spotted me, a welcome distraction from their everyday lives and they were very curious. Everyone wanted to know where I was from and asked me a million questions. Even those who did not speak were not any better as they stared at me continuously; it was very uncomfortable,' he said, grimacing.

Mike paused again as if to steel himself. 'Even in those overcrowded conditions, some people managed to read newspapers while others snacked or sang *bhajans* at the top of their voices. There were even hawkers who squeezed past with large wicker baskets! People just talked and talked and it was so intrusive and loud that I thought my head would explode. But finally, I reached Churchgate and got off.'

Mike finished recounting and looked at me with an exasperated expression. I smiled to make him feel more at ease, but I knew that now, after he had had a few days to digest the whole experience and calm down a bit, I had to make him understand certain things about it to help him get over it.

I could also see now how Mike had had an unpleasant walk to the station and a difficult train journey, but his extreme reaction was a bit of a surprise. Our mind tends to attach undue value to unpleasant events and provoke extreme decisions and behaviour.

Who decides our state of mind? We often carry animosity and hatred towards people because we have had a negative experience with them in the past. Don't you think life is too short to remain in an angry or unpleasant state, even temporarily, let alone for longer periods of time?

I wanted Mike to realize that his response to a bad experience was extreme, to say the least. But I knew that a direct counter-explanation wouldn't get through to him, rattled as his mind was by the journey. After all, the mind's job is to keep us safe, so it perceives difficult experiences as threats and tries to figure out ways to eliminate them. Thus, much of our anxiety and rash decisions are the result of an overzealous mind trying to protect us. But this protection often shields us from experiences that are more than necessary for us to grow. An overly protective mind hinders self-introspection. The answers to many of our problems lie in self-introspection but we hardly take the time needed to observe ourselves and our thoughts, emotions, responses and behaviour.

'Mike, you could have gotten kurtas and handicrafts in Santacruz. Why did you go all the way to Kala Ghoda to get these things? And that too alone?' I asked, trying to distract him from his recollections and further get to the bottom of things.

'Maa, my friend and classmate John had been there a few days ago. I liked the kurtas he bought from Kala Ghoda, so I went there as well,' he answered.

'Oh! So even John went to Kala Ghoda. How was his experience there?' I asked.

'I don't know, Maa. I never asked. It would probably have been the same,' Mike replied.

An inkling of an idea began to form in my mind. If it worked, Mike would see just how extreme our reactions can be to a *single bad experience.*

'Mike, can you and John meet me at 8.00 a.m. tomorrow?'

'Um, yes,' he said, unsure of what to expect.

'Good. Go rest now and I will see you both tomorrow,' I said.

Mike nodded, bid me goodbye and left the room.

The next morning, I woke up at 5.00 a.m. as usual and went about my normal morning routine of walking and doing my yoga *sadhana.* This is something I never miss. Even on the busiest of days, taking at least 5–10 minutes for my body is always a priority. No excuses to skip the morning yoga routine! After enjoying this routine and going over some of the other morning duties, I was ready to oversee my 7.30 a.m. teacher-training class. I take great joy and pride in observing the physical and mental progress of my students during the course and this morning was no different. Just as I finished my class, John walked into the room with a smile on his face. A smile is such a precious thing a person can wear! Carrying a smile has the power to positively impact you and the people around you.

A thirty-year-old mechanical engineer from France, John was soft-spoken, calm and friendly. Attentive and astute in class, he was loved by students and staff alike.

'Pranaam Maa,' John greeted me softly.

'Namaste John, how were your classes?'

'They went well. I really enjoyed the philosophy we are taught,' he replied enthusiastically.

'Good,' I said, smiling as well; his contagious smile had infected me.

'I'm here because Mike told me you wanted to meet me.'

'Yes, how is he? He seems a little worried,' I inquired.

'Maa, he is perturbed. He had a bad time travelling to Kala Ghoda. I heard he's considering quitting the course. It's surprising that he would think about leaving such a beautiful place,' said John and his brow furrowed fleetingly considering such a possibility but then finding his contagious smile again.

I nodded, acknowledging John's appreciative praise. The Yoga Institute had always been a home away from home for most of our students. Very rarely did anyone quit our course unless it was a real personal emergency. People felt close to home, to nature and their real selves here. For many, the institute offered beauty, joy, hope and peace. Yet Mike wanted to leave.

Do you have a Mike in you? Somewhere Mike reminds us of a part of ourselves—a part that makes us quit our goals, career, or relationship at the hint of the slightest difficulty. A part that fails to recognize the blessings in what we have chosen to quit. Do we really ever self-introspect on what we leave behind with every decision we take?

Just then Mike entered with a frown plastered on his face. I looked at the two of them, the smiling face and the frowning face right next to each other!

'Namaste Maa,' he said, huffing and panting.

'Namaste Mike, how was your morning?' I asked as the student sat down in front of me.

'It was okay,' he replied hesitantly. The worry in his voice and anxiety on his face was evident. I turned to John.

'So, John, can you tell us how your trip to Kala Ghoda went?' I looked at him expectantly.

Mike also turned to face John, expecting a similar version to what his experience had been.

'I had an amazing day,' John replied to Mike's utter shock. 'But Maa, it was a little tough for me too,' he added, almost as a consolation to Mike and giving him a quick glance.

John continued, 'It was a beautiful day. I walked out of the campus gates and the streets were full of people. Children played with each other, shouting with joy. Stray dogs jumped around them excitedly, as if they were best friends, often joining a game of cricket as an extra fielder. As I walked, people waved and talked to each other from homes on opposite ends of the street—people who seemed to have lived together for generations and shared the good and the bad, the joys and the sorrows. They were people who seemed like would never know how debilitating loneliness is, surrounded as they were by this gigantic display of care, love and friendliness. I have also become a big fan of the flower market, the fruit market and I'm even friends with some of the vendors now. While walking down the street, I enjoyed the fragrances of the flowers and fruits. It also never ceased to amaze me how cows majestically sun themselves in the middle of the street! Imagine this happening in France. Crows swooped down to steal a meal or two from unsuspecting people. People worshipped old, sturdy trees—common life was so intricately woven with nature! There was such closeness between people and the natural world despite Mumbai being one of the busiest and most crowded metropolises in the world.' He paused in thought.

'What of the piles of garbage and the spittle on the walls?' I asked.

'Maa, there was so much human energy, so much connection, so much life on the streets that the background faded into a distance,' said John.

'And the station, the train . . .?' I wanted to know John's full experience.

John inhaled audibly. 'That part of the travel was a little difficult, especially boarding the train since I travelled during peak hours.'

Mike clapped in triumph. 'That's what I said!'

John laughed and added enthusiastically, 'But now I think I can board any train in the world! I've learned a new skill. Boarding a Mumbai local train is indeed a skill and anyone who has mastered it is no less than Spiderman.'

He thumped his chest, not unlike a superhero, I thought to myself. Mike looked from my face to John's and then again at mine. But slivers of meaning had begun to creep into his worried, anxious mind.

'The people on the train were so loving,' John continued, reliving his experiences and making us a part of it. 'They were kind and helpful throughout, answering the questions I had about my destination and the many things I saw on the way from the train window. They even made sure I had a window seat! I truly felt like a celebrity, getting bombarded with questions and some people even trying to shake hands with me. It was a new and unexpected experience.'

The silence in the room was pregnant with meaning. John and I turned to face Mike. His face was full of thought but unlike before, it was not contorted with anxiety and unease.

'I understand. I think . . . I see now,' Mike offered tentatively. I could see he was still struggling to grasp the story John had narrated, so I decided to help him along a little.

'Mike, you had one bad day. One bad experience. It was difficult, I understand. But does it make sense to quit your course because of a bad day?' I asked.

Is It Easier to Quit or to Persist?

How many of us quit a job, give up on goals, or break off a relationship because of one small event or a single bad day? We tend to give the small and big occurrences of our life equal weightage in the way we think about them. Our responses to the small-scale, microcosmic events are, in fact, the best tools we can use to comprehend our thoughts and perceptions at subconscious levels since they possibly reflect our attitudes towards the outside world. Decisions, big or small, taken in frustration, anger, anxiety or stress are more likely to be destructive. It's best to refrain from even planning or speaking at such times.

Make It a Rule to Think, Act or Speak Only When You Are Calm

Mike seemed to have realized what we had been trying to explain. He spoke more to John about the rest of his experience and thought it over. After some soul-searching and a night of peaceful sleep, Mike rejoined the teacher-training course and life outside the campus with a new vigour.

> Never rush any decision.
>
> Often, we make hurried decisions after difficult experiences. Giving yourself time to recover from these experiences is vital. Time is healing. The quality of your decisions not only depends on how you take decisions but also on your state of mind while making it.

What can we learn from the two very different student's experiences? Are we more like Mike or John? And who do we want to be like? Let's review

Mike and John travelled on the same path, yet had extremely different experiences. Comparing their journeys shows us how different the same event can be. **The difference comes not from what is external, but from what is within us.** We all have a part within us that is like Mike and we all have a part in us that is John; the power lies in choosing to be a little more like John and a little less like Mike.

Don't you think we all experience life differently though we live in the same world? Having travelled across the globe,

I have noticed that people's issues, likes, dislikes and goals are similar, if not the same. Egos, attachments, relationship issues, health concerns and financial goals are all somewhat similar for many folks. Yet some experience each day as a gift while others experience it as a gruelling duel with their worst fears. This difference comes from what is within us and our attitudes towards events. Our reactions and responses towards the world outside determine the kind of life we lead more than anything else. We perceive events in our life as per our inherent or acquired tendencies. Some react quickly to events without a thought, whereas others pause, think, reflect and then respond. Some accept the struggles of life and face them, whereas others only crib and cry. Some treat their failures, even minor ones, as learning experiences whereas others give up even when confronted with the smallest of obstacles.

> We are all in the same boat of life but our perceptions decide whether we sink or swim.

How to Become a Positive and Cheerful Person

So, how do we reset our perceptions? How do we make each day less of a battle and more of a day full of learning and joy? How do we get to a right way of looking at things? For me, yoga as a philosophy had guided me to make right choices in life. Let's take a yogic look at three zones in Mike and John's journey:

1. The Street
2. The Railway Station
3. The Train

1

The Street

See both, good and bad, but stay close to the good.

Try to see both the good and bad parts of the situation but orient yourself towards the good. In life, if you look too closely or critically at something, you will only notice the worst in everything. As Oscar Wilde said, a cynic is one who knows the price of everything and the value of nothing.

Our anxiety-driven, survival-obsessed mind has conditioned us to be constantly critical, dissatisfied and blind to all that is good. **Finding faults is too easy for the mind.** You don't have to make an effort; it comes naturally to most of us since we've conditioned ourselves to think in this manner.

However, you must train your mind to see the positive side of everything as well. It needs time and determination. You don't have to make an effort to fall, but you do have to make an effort to rise. Similarly, look hard enough to see the better part of the situation.

'But if a flaw is a flaw, how can I ignore it? It needs to be addressed, right?' you may ask.

Yes, but you don't have to ignore it! You can acknowledge the flaw and act upon it. But you should not let it **influence your experience. It should be just like a small pinch, such as when a mosquito bites you.** You don't get stressed or depressed for a single mosquito bite, right? Your feelings, emotions should be based on the positives around things.

What about things that do not have a positive side to them? For example, suffering from a deadly disease or someone cheating innocent people? What could be positive about someone not fulfilling their assigned duties?

There are things that should never even happen; things that are wrong or unjust. Someone suffering a grave disease is unfair. Corruption and manipulation are unacceptable. It's hard to see the good side of such circumstances. Yet, even such situations offer you an opportunity to learn from them. Being sick teaches us to care for our body; cheating and manipulation offer the gift of wisdom and experience to the naïve. The laziness of those who shirk their work allows us the opportunity to set standards for ourselves.

You may have tried practising the positivity exercise I mentioned earlier. 'But what if I don't find any positive in a day?' you may ask.

It is a matter of practice. The more you start observing things in general, the more you will find the positive also. For example, wouldn't you say that as long as you have air to breathe and the earth to walk on, you'll always have at least two positive things in a day? The rest, as the bard said, lies in the eyes of the beholder.?

Initially, pinpointing the positive aspects in your life may seem like trying to see things in a dark room. The eyes strain to see anything at all but gradually, our sight adjusts and things begin to come into focus. Similarly, the more you **learn to train your mind** to notice the positive parts, the more they will appear to you. Noticing more of them is just an indication of an individual's internal progress—**the beginning of resetting your perception.**

Is it like the famous analogy of the half-full glass? Focusing on the part that is full? The idea is to **see everything; to see all the petals of the kailashpati flower, to see the empty part and the full part of the glass and the glass itself. One has to perceive both the good and the bad but the bad should not decide your state of mind, it should never be allowed to affect your mind. Your state of mind should be rooted in the positive part.**

2

The Railway Station

When feeling stuck, patience will give you the much-needed learning attitude.

Seeing different perspectives but choosing to focus on the good is essential for resetting our perception. However, nothing can be reset if we feel stuck, as Mike did at the railway station. The second zone in Mike and John's journey addresses this crucial issue: the feeling of being stuck. When Mike couldn't board five or six trains, he felt stuck; stuck because he wasn't getting where he wanted to be at the pace he wanted to. Don't we all experience this? When we don't get admission to a college of our choice, if we don't get the job in a company we want or married at the age we want—we feel stuck in life, like we are not where we should be. Or sometimes, we want to progress financially in our profession and when that doesn't happen, we feel trapped. In short, many times when we want to attain or achieve something and it doesn't happen, we feel helpless and/or dejected.

So when we are stuck, should we just give up on ourselves, our goals? We generally want to give up when like Mike, we operate from a place of apprehension and inexperience. Mike did not have the required experience to board a train in Mumbai; his inexperience caused repeated failure, which in turn added to his frustration during the trip to Kala Ghoda. Thus, when he had to wait; he was agitated and felt helpless.

However, all he needed to do was pause, observe and learn as John did. John noticed that there was a lot of pushing and shoving to get onto the train, but was fascinated by how anybody managed to board an already crowded train; yet so many managed! He observed how people did it and decided to look for a man with an office bag because he was more likely to be a daily passenger—a pro at boarding the train. John really wanted to learn the skill and observed a few office-goers board. He let two trains pass and as the third one arrived, he stood prepared behind a man with a briefcase. He even kept one hand gently over the man's back and followed him into the train. If Mike had had a similar learning attitude, then he would have been able to progress quickly. But his impatience and frustration clouded his observations and eventually his learning. A brief pause and some patience would have helped him learn how to get on the train. **A state of intermission is essential for a learning attitude.**

Sometimes, when we are stuck, all we need to do is take a breather to observe and learn from others. Learning from others doesn't make us small. In fact, one becomes wise and matures quickly if we have the eye to learn from other people and challenging situations. Being stuck either in a relationship or profession and being unable to move ahead only means that there is some kind of inexperience or apprehension that we can combat by gaining more insight into the matter.

Using Pauses—the Least Reinforcing Scenario (LRS)

There are certain methods of mental training that may serve as a good example at this point. The Least Reinforcing scenario (LRS), for instance, is used to train animals to perform certain feats in the circus or any other entertainment shows. What is it exactly? Whenever an animal makes a mistake during the training, the trainer stops, doesn't move, pausing for 3 seconds. This brief pause is enough to communicate to the animal that it is not supposed to repeat the mistake. It also communicates to the animal that it has made a mistake that it should correct. The pause acts not just as a communication tool but also as a space for the animal to observe and learn.

How many times do we feel tired and exhausted just in the middle of the day? **But have you ever paused, at that point, to understand what is it that you are doing wrong or where you are going wrong?** Mostly, we do not pause and take the time to learn from our mistakes. We continue repeating the same mistakes again and again every day, leading to issues such as health problems and failures in our life activities.

Are you repeating your mistakes or learning from them?

Another example to consider is a personal one, regarding a lady I know who broke her arm thrice while trying to reach a container on a high kitchen shelf. How? She used a stool, but it toppled and she broke her arm. Yet, she broke her arm again after a year, trying to use the same stool to reach for the same container! And a year later, she broke her arm again, using the same stool.

She didn't learn from the same mistake thrice! Don't you think we too make the same mistakes again and again in our life when we argue with our spouse for the same chore or when we overspend or over-eat again and again? Why do people fail to follow New Year's resolutions? It is because they do not learn from the failure of earlier resolutions. Developing a learning attitude becomes crucial for our happiness. If you genuinely want to develop a learning attitude within yourself, you must begin by taking a brief pause when you are in trouble, in pain, in a stressful or a clueless state, to self-reflect. When inventing the lightbulb, Thomas Alva Edison failed 1000 times and he simply learnt 999 ways of how to not approach the problem. What we do not acknowledge in this story is his patience after every failure. Every time he failed, he patiently tried to learn anew. If he had not been patient, he would have given up on his dream, there would not have been a lightbulb! Similarly, to bring light into our life, patience is indispensable.

Be patient, learn from others and from challenging situations and make sure not to repeat the same mistake again and again. We can rewire our thoughts to learn from every moment in our life. **Be patient—observe—learn.**

3

The Train

Develop a yogic attitude with *Maitri*, *Mudita*, *Karuna* and *Upeksha*

The difference between Mike and John's encounters on the train lies in the level of patience both individuals had and the significance of having a 'learning attitude'.

Mike was annoyed by people's behaviour. He disliked having to answer their intrusive questions. There was no privacy or sense of boundary. John, on the other hand, felt like a celebrity on the crowded train. People were very helpful, loving and caring. He thoroughly enjoyed talking to them and even made some new friends.

The people talking to Mike might not have intended to annoy him. They might simply have been trying to get to know him, where he is from, if he was finding it easy to settle down or so on.

That was affection. John saw that love in them. Hence, he too participated in the conversation with love. It is very easy to be distant and cold, but this only results in alienation and crippling loneliness.

Often, we are conditioned to think of people with suspicion or mistrust. Then, it is difficult to have an attitude of implicit trust and acceptance towards complete strangers.

Thus, we develop an attitude of mistrust. Your attitude is the lens through which you perceive the world. So when you have an attitude of mistrust, you cannot perceive anything as worthy of your confidence. Thus, an attitude reset is fundamental to 'resetting perception'.

Sometimes, all we must do is find joy in everyday things—like climbing stairs for example. In a social experiment, a big car company transformed the stairs in of a subway station in Stockholm, Sweden into working piano keys with the aim of motivating commuters to take the stairs rather than the escalator. When people stepped on the stairs, each step emitted a different musical note. This introduced an element of child-like joy and fun in their daily routine. The experiment worked out: people enjoyed playfully climbing the stairs. And the usually popular escalator was almost deserted when people started having fun on the stairs. What was once cumbersome became enjoyable and it helped people become more physically active as well. So it's all a matter of perception.

What does this example show us? Something as simple as the concept of fun can be the key to changing one's behaviour. That even mundane things can bring us joy; we just have to discover the joy in the everyday moments of life.

How can we put this attitude into practice? Next time you 'have to' do something, instead of doing it grudgingly and without much thought, think about how you 'get to' do it and how it is a privilege. For example, if you are not too fond of household chores—dusting, washing the dishes or cleaning the floors or the bathrooms—think about how lucky you are to have so many shelves for your possessions, beautiful dishes to wash, so much floor space to mop and a nice bathroom to use. It should be a joy to keep all these things in working condition and sparkling clean. If you need yet another example of how to change one's perception, read the famous excerpt in Mark Twain's *The Adventures of Tom Sawyer* where Tom makes painting a fence seem so attractive that his friends practically fight each other for the joy of wielding the paintbrush for a few strokes.

In terms of our relationship with others, Yoga philosophy suggests that your attitude to any individual should consist of either one of the following four values:

1. *Maitri*
2. *Mudita*
3. *Karuna*
4. *Upeksha*

Maitri: Friendly Attitude. Maintain a friendly attitude towards everyone, even strangers. John didn't know his co-passengers on the train, yet he was friendly towards them which made his journey enjoyable. Mike's mistrust only made things worse for him. If life was a train journey, would you like it to be like John's journey or Mike's journey? The former requires maitri. Would being friendly to people who were curious about him and wanted to know about his home country really have harmed Mike? Unfriendliness is often the consequence of insecurity and worry. A *maitri bhava* can help you reduce all these unnecessary emotions in your life.

Mudita: Possessing an attitude of happiness, on a tangible and practical basis. Be happy for yourself and happy that you woke up to another day. Tomorrow is not a given! Be happy even if you have a job you dislike because even then your life has its *positive points,* for example a healthy body, a loving family or other boons. Even the job you may dislike supports you financially. So celebrate yourself and your life. Mudita also involves being happy seeing others succeed or grow. It discourages feelings of envy and jealousy towards others. When you cultivate mudita and feel joy and peace for the success of other people, you are constantly in a state of calm.

Karuna: Empathy. Put yourself in another person's shoes to understand what they experience. This helps us understand people better. Try to put yourself in your spouse's place when you repeatedly fail to prioritize your relationship or in your manager's place if you think a particular deadline is harsh. In relationships, we sometimes fail to understand what the other person is going through and that lack of sensitivity leads to conflict. For instance, parents might impose too many restrictions on their child without realizing what they are going through. For instance, children often shout and scream or lash out when they feel unseen and unheard. In such situations, empathizing with your child allows you to understand that your child feels unseen. Gently place your hand on your child's shoulder and tell them that you see and understand them and that they do not have to shout for your attention. Karuna can form the basis for a strong and loving bond between you and your child, spouse, colleagues and friends. Experiencing the world as another person will help you cultivate the right attitude towards them and reset your perception of them.

Upeksha: Non-discrimination. Don't judge people for their money, their social standing, their habits, their emotions, or their preferences. We often make the mistake of valuing people for their money or social standing. These assumptions are as frivolous as the speculations people made about the value of pepper in the golden age of the spice trade or the early value of VCRs. Instead, value loyalty, value those who stand by you even when you are unsuccessful, value those who care enough to be honest with you and give you opinions that may be difficult to hear but ultimately, are the best for you.

Developing such attitudes is important for your peace and for you to have a rich, rewarding life. Excessive isolation and seclusion can take a toll on the mind; it is healthy to seek out meaningful connections with others and form relationships. When we connect with people, either directly or indirectly, many of them may not behave or act in the way we want. But if our attitude towards them contains one of the four qualities discussed above, we can reset our perception of them, rework our relationships with them and reform the very experiences of our life.

Resetting perception saves your energy; your *prana*. It helps you avoid overthinking and exhaustion. To summarize, what exactly do you need to do in order to reset your perception? Remember Mike and John's journey to Kala Ghoda; remember what the three metaphors teach us:

- The Street: See both: Good and Bad but stay close to the good.
- The Railway Station: The feeling of being stuck : Be patient, observe and learn.
- The Train: Develop a yogic attitude: Maitri, Mudita, Karuna and Upeksha

And if all this is a little too much, remember the little squirrel on the kailashpati tree. Be like that. Enjoy the beauty of the world around you a little more and worry a little less about everything else.

THREE

Reset Your Social Life

'No man is an island, entire of itself;
Every man is a piece of the continent, a part of the main.'
—John Donne

The train chugged slowly into Indore station and I felt the city's gentle breeze on my face. It was almost as if the city was welcoming me back—a grandmother anxiously and lovingly waiting for her grandchild. I have always loved the night train from Mumbai to Indore. It seemed as if in one night, the train moved through time, taking me back towards the oldest, fondest memories of my childhood. These memories were of Indore; old, regal Indore and young, vibrant Indore. Indore always made me feel as if my distant childhood was just around the corner—near enough that if I just reached my hand out of the window, I could almost touch it. I felt like I was a child again and all the grey and silver on my head was simply some false shadow beyond age and time.

'Hansaji, you must have so many memories of Indore,' remarked my travelling companion, Rohita, as she took in all the sights and sounds of the bustling railway station.

'Yes, Rohita,' I said with a smile as my mind wandered back to what the city meant to me.

Indore has always had a special place in my heart. After all, I spent countless summer holidays in the city. So many years ago, as a child, the city's palaces, the bazaars and the gardens had been the centre of many of my adventures. I remembered the countless afternoons of hide and seek, the thrill of running wild through the mango orchards, swinging so high that I thought I would touch the clouds and the many nights we spent gazing at the stars. I couldn't help but smile at myself and at the power of memories of old playmates and playthings. Memories sometimes play hide and seek with us; hiding old friends and hiding the people who gave us good and bad experiences. But we always manage to seek out the ones that are special to us; much like how this sudden trip had brought out the memories of my childhood to me. What we did when we were young finds a special place in our memories, irreplaceable as childhood is in our hearts! It's best to give a special place only to the joyful memories. Life will be happier that way.

The train came to a halt and so did the gentle musings of my mind, albeit grudgingly. There was an explosion of activity all around me. I sat back to enjoy the show. People rushed to get to the door with their luggage. Children squealed in excitement and anticipation. On the platform, vendors peddling tea and savouries screeched at the top of their voices. People thronged to them to savour their morning cuppa; some had the distinct expressions of getting their morning fix. Seeing people take hot cups of tea to their families waiting in the train carriages was such a touching display of care and affection, yet went so often unnoticed. A smile warmer than the cups of tea being served on a railway station in the heart of India made its way to my face. I have always loved travelling by train. It is surprising how quickly we manage to talk to strangers on the train—giving and sharing life advice, discussing family problems, or commenting on the state of events with absolute trust. Travelling on trains in India has taught me that we, as a people, trust implicitly. That is why we don't seem to mind talking so unguardedly to the unfamiliar people sitting next to us on the train. It is this peculiar quality that sometimes turns our co-passengers into friends and allies. I even knew of a few people who had set up marriage alliances on these journeys. Such is the way of life on the rails! Well, at least before mobiles phones slowly crept into our lives. Nowadays, people are glued to their screens, rather than enjoying the live screen telecast of existence that plays out in trains.

Meanwhile, scores of coolies thronged towards the compartments of my train, squeezing their way through the crowd at the door. They yelled and scurried through at lightning speeds, trying their best to secure customers. I have always marvelled at how they competed fiercely with each other every day for the same customers and the same gains but did so with a sense of brotherhood and were never against each other. This was true for the city as a whole too. Everyone worked towards their goals competitively, yet there were some invisible threads that seemed to connect everybody in the city. These threads that made the whole city throb with life when there was a festival to be celebrated or a cricket match victory to be deified. Maybe, I speak with a slight bias for my old friend, Indore, but our friends always manage to evoke special feelings in us. What can one do?

Just then I saw the face of my old student, Professor Vimal Nath. He was trying to squeeze through the crowded compartment in the direction of my seat. Professor Nath was erudite, accomplished, well-respected and had many talents but navigating through the crowds of an Indian train was not one of his many skills. I suppressed a smile as the learned professor was unceremoniously spat out by the wave of people trying to exit the compartment. A man of books, Vimal sometimes forgot even now, that the world of people worked a little differently. Now slightly dishevelled, the professor smiled sheepishly at me from the platform. Kamala, his wife and I rolled our eyes at each other over his valiant attempts.

The sudden trip to Indore was all thanks to my old friends Vimal and Kamala Nath. Dear, old Vimal had been conferred a prestigious award for distinguished service and exemplary leadership. Kamala and Vimal had been elated when they discovered that I would be presenting the award and had insisted that I stay with them for this trip. They had been adamant and refused to take no for an answer and so, I agreed. Vimal and Kamla were accompanied by many of my other students who had heard that I would be coming to Indore. Most of them had insisted that I stay with them for my stay in Indore but Vimal had managed to keep them all at bay. But they had insisted that they would come to receive me at the station. Their eager, happy faces filled me with pleasure since I was seeing them all after such a long time. Everyone waved excitedly at me and I waved back.

Slowly the crowd in my compartment thinned and Vimal and Kamala helped us get out. Despite the crowded station, we managed to make our way out of there and were soon comfortably ensconced in the car, driving towards their house.

Sometime later, I was refreshed and situated in the living room of the Naths, enjoying their gracious hospitality. I believe that the hospitality and graciousness with which we treat our guests does us a lot of good. Firstly, it makes us consider things outside of ourselves and our minds. Secondly, just the act of doing something nice to make someone feel welcome and comfortable unleashes a barrage of positive emotions and joy in us. Finally, in welcoming someone into our house, we welcome their presence, their wisdom and with it, the possibility of friendship and support. Culturally too, the Indian emphasis on hospitality is entrenched within all of us. *Athithi devo bhava*—the guest is like a god—is a very real philosophy for us.

The Naths too have always taken this adage quite literally—the wide array of food they had placed before me would have been a meal fit for the pickiest of gods!

Kamala and Vimal beamed at me. 'We weren't sure what you would like, so we bought a little of everything from Sarafa,' said Kamala.

'It looks like you got the entire Sarafa market for me, Kamala!' I said, wondering how they expected me to eat so much. Their giant table was creaking under the weight of everything they had put on it.

Sarafa market is very special to Indore, because of its late-night, street food market. Sarafa comes alive under the stars every night and offers visitors an array of *chaat, namkeen* and every other conceivable combination of snacks. Some people even say that Sarafa has as many types of dishes as the stars in the night sky.

'Hansaji, would you like something else?' asked Professor Nath, carrying in a tray of hot herbal tea from the kitchen. Over the years, Vimal had become specialized in the making of herbal tea. Anyone who visited the Naths was sure to be treated to the marvellous machinations of Vimal's herbal tea-making.

'Making the perfect cup of herbal tea is an art,' Vimal always said. But he never revealed the secret behind his art—he was a little more than protective of his knowledge. Kamala always teased him about how he had perhaps stolen the recipe, but he remained tight-lipped about it despite his wife's many snubs. Kamala and Vimal were always playful with each other and their relationship was full of joy and friendship. This friendship, I believe, was the cornerstone of their long and happy marriage.

'Have a mathri, Hansaji,' said Vimal, putting the plate right under my nose. Flaky, crunchy and lightly spiced mathris are a delicacy in Indore. No host worth their salt would skip out on serving mathris. Kamala lathered hers with a generous dose of tangy mango pickle, placed it in her mouth and crunched. I swallowed as the combination of mathri and pickle did not exactly fit into my satvik diet. But the look on Vimal's face was so entreating that it would take a heart of stone to refuse him. I gingerly took a mathri and bit into it as Vimal and Kamala beamed their 100-watt smiles at me.

Sometimes, life is like this. You do little things you don't like because they cause big things you love. The big thing here was the happiness on their faces and that happiness made it worthwhile. When we make such tiny adjustments to our social lives, we are oiling the screws and hinges of our relationships with others. If we neglect to do this, our social lives will become like creaky old doors that struggle to open smoothly and create hindrances whenever someone tries to enter our lives. Welcome those who come in with a smile, let go of those who leave with warmth, and you will be surrounded by good friends and companions for the rest of your life.

Rohita seemed to have become a new fan of Vimal's herbal tea as well. As she relished another sip, she turned to me and asked, 'Hansaji, Professor Nath seems to be your student. How did you two meet?'

I picked up my cup of tea and looked at Vimal and Kamala. Taking a sip, I explained, 'It was many years ago when we first met. Professor Nath was a fresh-faced doctoral graduate who had recently begun working in a prestigious college. Right, Vimal?'

Vimal nodded in agreement. 'It was during the annual break in college. I had just enrolled myself in a course with The Yoga Institute in Mumbai.'

'Oh! Did you take some time off to go to Mumbai, Vimal?' Kamala asked.

'Yes! It was quite long ago. Nothing was digital. Only government offices had computers back then. Everything was offline, especially courses. Right, Hansaji?'

I nodded in agreement, 'Those were different days, Kamala. Everything was physical and nothing was digital. Life was slow and we all went with the flow. And Vimal had been a different man too—ahead of his time with all his ideas and plans. And he had none of his special tea-making skills!'

Vimal smiled, but his smile did not reach his eyes. A faint expression of hurt crossed his rotund face when he thought of that time, so long ago. He began to tell them his tale of loss and suffering.

'I had been suspended from my job and since I was still in my probation-period I could also be fired.' Vimal said looking at me.

'What! Suspended? You? You are one of the most popular professors on campus and have had a thirty-year-long, distinguished career in this college!' Kamala exclaimed in disbelief.

'I was popular then as well, Kamala but only with the students. My work-life was a complete mess. I had managed to alienate everyone, from the director to the peon and as a result, was about to be fired from my dream job. And I would have been fired too, had I not joined the course at The Yoga Institute,' Vimal whispered.

Kamala looked stunned.

I placed my cup of tea on the table. 'In the course too, Vimal was not making any friends. He did everything perfectly: the asanas, the kriyas; he followed the satvik diet properly and yet, not even the tutors developed a fondness for him,' I glanced at the two of them, remembering Vimal during the course just as though it were yesterday.

'I liked to believe I was an acquired taste in those days,' Vimal said sheepishly. Kamala ignored him and looked at me.

I continued, 'Vimal always came to class before anyone else, even the teachers. He took his place at the very front of the class. He never looked at anyone or smiled at any of his course mates. He looked on ahead, determined to prove that he was the best of the best!'

Vimal nodded in agreement with me, but Kamala had her mouth open like a goldfish and blurted, 'But he smiles even at random strangers now! He asks them how their day has been, requests them to be detailed and really listens.'

Kamala couldn't believe that the man she had married could have been so different at that time. It was difficult for her to accept that jovial, easy-going Vimal could have once been a much-misunderstood man. The surprise on her face was evident to Vimal and me. I said, 'Vimal never did anything untoward or palpably wrong. But we began to receive requests from teachers and students, requesting we shift him to another batch for no clear reason apart from how he just made them feel uncomfortable in ways that they couldn't explain.'

'And that's how I ended up meeting Hansaji in her office one summer evening, certain that everyone and everything in life was unfair to me and that I was going to be ousted from The Yoga Institute too, despite trying my best in the course. It felt as if my bad luck from Indore had followed me to Mumbai,' said Vimal.

'Well, then what happened?' Kamala was eager for the story to continue.

'Hansaji had different plans for me. I realized later that she did not intend to be unfair to me, nor was she going to throw me out of the course. Well, not right away. Maybe she was waiting till I managed to anger the entire class with my behaviour!' he joked lamely.

Nobody laughed. Comedy was clearly not his forte even now.

I said, 'That day, I saw an educated young man who had the world before him. But I also sensed that he seemed to have an attitude of bearing the weight of it as well on his shoulders. I offered him a seat.'

'Namaste Hansaji,' Vimal greeted me politely as he sat, I felt as if his greeting had no warmth. I slowly began to see what might be going on. But I also sensed that it would not be easy to make him see what everyone else felt. Nonetheless, I was interested in seeing how this meeting would play out and asked him how the course was going.'

'The course is satisfactory, Hansaji, but . . .'

'But?' I asked.

Vimal was surprised that I wanted to hear more from him, but he did not hesitate to share his unfiltered views. 'The other students expect me to talk to them, chat about random things like movies and heroes and socialize with them. Despite the programme's emphasis on satvik meals, some of them even suggested that we go out and enjoy some tea and vada pavs after the session!'

Vimal, I realized, was attending the course but he was yet to understand the essence of it. Asanas, kriyas and a satvik diet were part of the course, but fundamentally, it was about something greater. It was about the value of little things, about the value of the single moment. Yoga was not some movement towards a grand climax; it was about weaving joy and contentment into every small aspect of your life. I would have to make sure that he understood that! I smiled at him.

'Is that all, Vimal?'

I felt a strain of emotions—difficult and choking, enter his voice while his eyes began to moisten.

'The . . .' he whispered. 'The college . . . in college, in Indore,'
he trailed.

'What happened in Indore, Vimal?' I prodded calmly.

He looked at me, visibly uncomfortable and broke down.
He seemed lost. I knew that nothing else would come out of this
evening. I managed to calm him and got him to have a light meal
before sending him off to bed.

The next morning, I sat in the gazebo with Pratik, a
student of mine. The gazebo was a favourite spot of mine
on the campus as it had a moat of water running around
it. I loved sitting in the gazebo and dipping my feet in the
water; it reminded me of dipping my feet in the playful rivers
near my grandmother's house. I think I imbibed my sense
of play from them; it's a priceless gift that has always helped
me through life's challenges. I have just always known, in my
heart, that flowing water can wash away all that is stagnant
and no longer serves you. That morning, I was trying to teach
this to Pratik, who was another student working so hard that
he had affected his health badly. Pratik was very dedicated
and serious. I needed to remind him of the importance of
having a sense of lightness and playfulness in life. I had to
make him understand that if something happened to him, the
office would find a replacement for him in six months. Pratik,
like many of us, needed to grasp that **work is just a part of our**
life, it is not all of our life.

As Vimal walked up to us, Pratik got up, nodded to me,
then to Vimal and left.

'Namaste Hansaji,' Vimal said gravely.

I wondered why he was so serious on such a bright and
beautiful day when the sun shone gently, the birds chirped

merrily and the squirrels danced vigorously. When we greet someone, it should be a communication of a heartfelt joy of meeting another person. Nowadays, so many of us suffer from loneliness and isolation. These problems crop up because we forget the simple basics of etiquette that are passed down to us in our culture. Culturally, we are so attuned to joy and celebration that we make even a simple greeting a matter of joy. But Vimal was so solemn, that it seemed as though he was completely blind to all that was living around him in his pursuit of some outward goal. He seemed to remind me of people who are often accomplished and sometimes successful, but very rarely happy or satisfied. Nonetheless, I had to respond to Vimal's prim and proper greeting.

'Namaste, Vimal,' I replied with a smile.

'Hansaji, you give up so much of your time and energy for others. How does a person of your stature manage to do this and that too for regular people like us?' he asked.

I could also see why Vimal's sense of righteousness had been making everyone around him uncomfortable. But before I could delve into that, I had to answer his question.

'Stature . . . Vimal? Stature . . .?' I said softly. 'The mighty banyan tree is large and may even cover acres and acres of land, but the slender guava tree or the waif-like *neem* may not take more than a few feet of ground. What makes you think there is any question of stature amongst them! They may seem different, one larger than the other, but that does not necessarily mean one is more important than the other!'

'But . . .but . . .' Vimal sputtered, at a loss of words.

'Vimal, have you seen how, despite its stature, the banyan is so alone in the forest and spread out over such a vast area that no other tree can grow near it? But the guava or the neem grows in the heart of the forest surrounded by other trees, plants and all that is living and thriving. Have you ever noticed how alone the banyan seems despite its majesty and stature?'

'A-alone? . . . Banyan . . . stature?' Vimal muttered.

'Aren't you also like the banyan, Vimal, upright, accomplished and righteous, but alone?' I suggested to the young professor from Indore.

Vimal seemed to be taken aback, indignant that someone would see through him and terrified about what would happen if nobody did. I sensed that this was his moment of vulnerability where he had let down his guard and seized it.

'What happened in Indore, Vimal?' I asked. 'What happened at the college in Indore?'

He looked straight at me, but I knew he did not see me; his mind was in Indore and poring over the many difficulties that life seemed to have heaped upon his young shoulders. Gradually, however, he began, 'I got my dream job as a lecturer in one of Indore's most prestigious colleges as soon as I finished my PhD. It was no small achievement, Hansaji. Most of my co-doctoral fellows are still struggling to find a job. However, I had top grades throughout and it was no surprise that I was selected for the position.'

His happiness and eagerness for his job shone through his eyes.

He continued, 'I was beyond myself with happiness. I had so many ideas for the department, so many changes for the curriculum, the teaching methodology, the research subjects and the corrections, I could teach them so much and I wanted my department to become the best in the country. I knew my department would soon attract international funding and research. I was ready to put my heart and soul into the job.'

'That did not work out so well, right?' I asked.

He nodded in agreement.

'What happened, Vimal?' I asked.

'I tried to tell everyone that what they were doing for so long was incorrect. That we had to change, change for the better of the department, the college! That we could produce world-class research and attract the best funding. But slowly, everyone began to ignore me and then most of them became positively antagonistic. I still cannot understand why! My ideas were so good that they would have taken the department to new heights,' he said, lamenting.

'So, you are facing challenges in working with your colleagues, is that it? I asked.

He said, 'At first, it was just my colleagues but slowly, even the management of the college began to resent me and my proposals. They said my proposals were not practical! I know it was really their unwillingness to change a system which worked perfectly well for them. They valued their comfort zone too much. This was not in the best interests of my department or college, so I confronted them and then, I even communicated my grievances to the higher authorities.'

'That was not a particularly smart thing to do, was it Vimal?' I asked.

He nodded. 'It wasn't. Once it was known that I had taken the matter forwards, I was the proverbial black sheep, an outcast in my department and college. Nobody would have anything to do with me. Supporting me or my proposals or even simply talking to me meant putting your career in jeopardy. My colleagues were more than happy with the state of things as they could now saunter back to their staid, conformist methods of working.'

'Well, that does not sound good, Vimal,' I said.

'It was not, Hansaji. Soon, the other members of the staff began to complain to everyone else that I was too aloof. Many of them were offended that I would not waste my time in idle gossip over tea and snacks. I don't approve of such things during working hours. I believe in being completely dedicated to the job. Others were offended that I would not attend events like weddings, or birthdays that they had personally invited me to. I believe that these celebrations are unimportant and waste a lot of money,' Vimal explained.

'So, you thought that spending some time talking to the people you work with or accepting their invitations to share in their celebrations and their joy was futile?' I asked in disbelief.

We all chase grand plans, have ambitions and desire greatness. But in doing so, we forget that the greatest things that happen to our lives are hidden in the smallest moments. That is a mistake we all make. He had missed out on so much vital human connection and bonding by keeping himself away from his colleagues, their joys and sorrows. **Remember, in life, there is no big without the small; there is no grand without the ordinary.** Think about it. It will come to you.

Vimal nodded in agreement. 'But that was not all, Hansaji. Slowly, my students were alienated from me as well. They used to love my lectures. But my department worked against me to assign the least number of classes to me and only on all the non-core subjects of the syllabus. I think the students somehow got the message that if any kind of closeness or appreciation for me was seen, it would affect their grades in other subjects. Since I was not allotted any of the elective subjects, my grades or courses had no real value. Slowly there was an irreparable breakdown between me and my students. They did not see any value in what I had to offer.'

'Which also effectively means the end of your academic career,' I remarked, getting a clearer idea of how things went wrong for the bright and dedicated Vimal.

'But Hansaji, that was not the reason for my immediate suspension. Despite the fact that I taught non-core subjects, I made it a point to push my students. I held them to standards of excellence. They began to resent my expectations of them. All kinds of complaints were lodged against me, from academic ones to complaints of impropriety and harassment. Finally, the Academic Committee and the Disciplinary Committee got involved. I was suspended. I lost everything that mattered the most to me,' he said, suppressing a sob.

I felt bad for the young man before me; genius or not, he was a little rough around the edges. While Vimal may have been a bit off in his approach, his intentions seemed genuine.

'What would you do, Hansaji, if you were in my place?' he asked.

'Vimal, life is not a quadratic equation that you will simply crack if you spend hours and hours working on it. In life, **evolution, not revolution, is the name of the game,**' I replied.

Vimal looked flabbergasted. If he were a cartoon character, he would be like one of those whose lower jaw drops completely to the floor and their mouth is wide open.

'Let's meet again tomorrow morning, Vimal. You will see things differently. I promise,' I said and walked away for another urgent counselling session. Out of the corner of my eye, I saw him rooted to the spot just as he was rooted to the mistakes that got him in this position in the first place.

'Evolution, not revolution,' I whispered to myself, as Vimal slowly disappeared out of my view.

The next morning, Vimal found me near the gazebo again. I could see he was trying hard to accept all that we had talked about yesterday.

'Namaste Hansaji,' he said. I noticed something new. Though still formal and stilted, his greeting had an almost hidden tone of warmth and joy to it. *Well, yesterday was not a complete washout*, I thought to myself.

'Namaste Vimal,' I said and smiled back. 'Would you like to try dipping your feet in the waters? They're very calming. They will wash away all your burdens.'

Suddenly, Vimal seemed extremely offended. 'No, Hansaji. My burdens are too heavy for this little stream,' he murmured.

'Vimal, we are not meant to live or work alone. Work and life go hand in hand."

'Hansaji, I joined this course to reset my work and life. I do not believe in new-age, wishy-washy philosophies that tell you not to compete or do your best in your workplace at any cost!' Vimal rasped.

'Vimal, yoga is completely committed to karma. Action is at the heart of yogic philosophy. It is rather incorrect view that Yoga cannot understand the competitive instincts of the modern workplace. As talented as you are, you will not succeed without learning to work with others,' I suggested.

'Work with others?'

He seemed lost. I decided to explain, 'See Vimal, here at the Yoga Institute, we have our own little secret to sort out work-related issues.'

'W-work-related issues . . .?' he stuttered.

'We call it the five-star method. Would you like to hear about it?' I asked.

He nodded with curiosity.

The Five-Star Method to Reset Your Work-Life

1. Recognize the importance of allies.

Do you remember Abhimanyu in the Mahabharata war? Abhimanyu knew how to enter the *chakravyuha*, a military formation, but his father, the warrior Arjuna, had not yet taught him the secret to getting out of it. Outside the chakravyuha and inside it Abhimanyu was a great warrior but outside he had allies; inside it he was alone.

There is a lot one can learn from this story. Specifically, it underlines the importance of allies. Credibility and competence can only get you so far. It is imperative that we recognize the worth of our interpersonal networks and connections. Vimal believed that his degrees and his academic achievements put him on a level where he did not need anyone else. He believed he was a world unto himself. But then, when that world caught fire, there was no one to help put out the flames. When Vimal's colleagues began to resent him, if he had had an ally amongst them, would he not have escaped his downward spiral completely? If Vimal had someone who could have pointed out to him the resentment and heartburn he was causing, if someone told him the error of his ways in annoying the management would a brilliant career have been threatened?

Remember this: Anyone who wants to be a successful leader, or simply good at their job, needs to recognize the importance of allies. Allies in the modern workplace serve a very crucial role. They speak for you in positions and situations that may not be accessible to you. They recognize your abilities and the value you add to the organization. But it's not a one-way street. **Recognize that forming allies relies on forming mutually beneficial ties.** The professional world is not an altruistic one. You must practically understand and accept its realities and try to work within the boundaries of ethics, with a spirit of goodwill. So understand that **no one will be your ally until you are theirs. It is a world of give and take; so participate in the world according to its rules.**

When it comes to understanding the true nature of allies, learn from the relationship between King Rama and Sugriva. Rama, the statesman and warrior prince, regained for Sugriva the kingdom of Kishkinda from his brother Vali. Sugriva, in turn, placed at Rama's disposal the use of the vast monkey army and the services of warriors like Jambavan, Angad and Hanuman. This teaches us the importance of having friends, relatives and social connections. We need our social network to function well not only professionally, but personally and emotionally as well. **Mutuality has been and will remain the essence of forming allies. Know this as you face your professional challenges and you will find that no mountain is too high for you.**

2. How to deal with politics

A major reason behind Professor Vimal's alienation and isolation in his workplace was his belief that his competence and credentials made him immune to office politics. One must understand that politics is a part and parcel of life. Instead of seeing it as something negative, think of it as a game. A game where everyone's ultimate objective is to win. So play, play with all your heart! Play with the subtleties of your mind. And play to win!

A workplace cannot be completely democratic or completely fair all the time as well. But you cannot be childish and expect it to. For instance, if you are playing hide-and-seek and you realize that the seeker is cheating, so you stop playing. If you do so, you lose by forfeit since the game will go on regardless. The trick is to beat the seeker at their own game. If something is not ideal, learn to not respond to it emotionally. Accept that a professional workplace is tuned to the needs of the organization and not to individual notions of ethics. Think of lawyers who represent criminals. They may personally believe that theft or murder is not right. But their profession and the law requires them to defend their client, who may have committed such acts, to ensure a fair trial. In defending their clients, they must participate in professional politics.

Recognize that an office or company offers you lessons on practicality. Going to work is not the same thing as going to school or college or getting your PhD. It's a completely different ballgame. For starters, you never know the question you need to answer. Every day is a new challenge and you will encounter new people, new situations and will need to innovate in the way you did the previous day. **Learning when to engage and disengage with office politics at the right time is an exercise in practical innovation and action.**

Dealing with politics in the workplace will give you an understanding of different kinds of knowledge. Take Vimal's example. Vimal realized that a college cannot be run by lecturers alone, however competent they may be. To be an organic whole, the college needs people with a diverse mix of skills that range from academic sharpness and administrative far-sightedness to financial acumen. This is true for any institution or organization, from small NGOs to the largest of MNCs.

Do not assume that only competence will make you successful or be the cause of your organization's success. Being well-versed with people skills is often at the heart of success.

People are everything! And if there are people, there will be politics. Don't run from it. Play with it.

3.   Try the Goldilocks method for workplace socializing

At the end of the day, you must realize and accept that any professional area is a community space, not an individual one. You cannot expect to work in an organization, office or company and have nothing to do with your colleagues. You cannot be an island in the workplace. This is applicable whether you're a freelancer, business owner, CEO or hospitality and housekeeping staff. It is vital that you cultivate the skill of socializing in the workplace.

Vimal pushed his colleagues away to a great degree when he refused to spend time with them over tea. This caused two major problems for Vimal's image with them. Firstly, he came across as a snob who thought he was better than the people around him. People generally tend to dislike snobs. When Vimal continued to work as his colleagues took their breaks; Vimal appeared like someone out to prove that he was a conscientious and dedicated worker while his colleagues were all slackers. We can all assume that nobody liked the way Vimal made them feel and he was gradually slowly pushed out of the office-circle as a result of this.

Secondly, Vimal's attitude made him look like a workaholic. Work is important, no doubt. But how you work is equally important; if not more important. Any work that is done should have a sense of purpose and satisfaction but most importantly a sense of play. Research has shown that teams, where leaders encourage recreational activities or group bonding beyond work hours, are more productive. On the flip side, group leaders who are strict disciplinarians and emphasize deadlines and results, usually receive subpar results from their teams. Vimal did not understand that breaks and friendly chit-chat could do far more for productivity as compared to sitting rigidly at his desk for hours. If nothing, such activities encourage a sense of companionship. **People tend to work better when they feel appreciated and like the people they work with.**

So, does this mean you spend all your time flitting from desk to desk and gossiping when you are supposed to be working? No, not unless you are looking for a way to get yourself fired. Socializing at the workplace is nothing short of an art and at the Yoga Institute, we refer to it as the Goldilocks way. It's simple really. Just as dear old Goldilocks didn't like the porridge to be too hot or too cold or the bed too hard or too soft, one must socialize not too much or too little at the workplace. **It must be done just right!**

When colleagues invite you for tea or coffee breaks with them, see if you can comfortably make it a part of your daily routine. Spending a few minutes getting to know the people you work with can hardly be considered a waste of your time. Now, if you don't like mingling every day, do it just once or twice a week. Sometimes, take the initiative and invite your colleagues out for tea. This way you won't seem like an indifferent snob but as someone who is a part of the team.

The same formula applies to social invitations. Never refuse them outright. Try to always show up and look happy for the joys of others. This will create in them a subconscious belief that you are on their side; they will like you more and appreciate working with you. **Remember, people work better when they like the people they are working with!**

Slowly, you may even overcome any personal aversions you may have to public gatherings or celebrations. You may even grow to like them and think of them as someone sharing the special moments of their life with you. **Start socializing in moderation, be Goldilocks and see where it takes you.**

4.   Be people-oriented rather than only process-oriented

Another major error Vimal made in his earnest endeavour to bring about changes in his college was that he was completely process-oriented! Vimal wanted to change everything—the evaluation system, the teaching methodology, the curriculum—all in one go! While he did a thorough analysis of what process would work and what would not, he forgot one tiny detail: it's about the people, not the process. This does not mean focusing solely on people's emotions in the workplace. After all, you are in a professional environment where you eventually must deliver on your goals. But remember that any change you wish to introduce should add value to the people who are a part of that organization, whether they are staff or patrons.

In Vimal's case, he pressed his students to perform well in their elective courses too, turning a blind eye to the added burden this would mean for them. Did his actions add value to his students or did they add value to his sense of self? This is where most of us go wrong. **We often believe that what we are doing is good for others, when it is actually only good for us.** If Vimal had simply paused to examine the effect of his actions on his students, he perhaps would not have alienated them as well. The same applies to his insistence that his colleagues adopt the changes he had suggested. His process may have been thorough, but he did not analyze how capable his colleagues were of adapting to his changes. Without a sense of readiness and acceptance about Vimal's plans, would have seemed threatening to them and their livelihoods. Their rejection of his ideas and Vimal's subsequent ostracism have their roots in the sense of insecurity that his process-oriented plans provoked.

I will again clarify that being people-oriented at the workplace in no way means taking responsibility for someone's emotions and feelings. But it does imply that you assess situations in an unbiased way as to how prepared people are for the process you are trying to introduce. A people-oriented approach makes one aware of the time and effort needed for new processes to take root. A people-oriented approach focuses on upskilling and upgrading people, making the new process more enabling and less endangering.

5. Try for evolution, not revolution, in life

Vimal never really appreciated the simplicity of the water that surrounded the gazebo, caught up as he was in the question of stature and uprightness. A rigid mind finds it exceptionally difficult to appreciate the finesse of flexibility. This was possibly a major reason his career was suffering.

Vimal might have had excellent ideas that would have projected his department to newer heights of success. But he forgot that ideas are one half of the game; the other half is people. Any idea, however profitable, has to be acceptable to the people you work with. If not, then the time for the idea has not come just yet.

So, do we give up on all our brilliant ideas because people might not agree with them? Of course not! If people did not come out with new ideas, we would still believe that the earth is flat and Newton wouldn't have discovered gravity. The forwards momentum of the human race depends on revolutionary ideas. But in the workplace, how you present these ideas is of vital importance. Present your ideas as a gentle evolution from the way things are rather than a disruptive revolution of the present order.

Revolutions are scary for most people as they challenge the scheme of events; events that people are comfortable with. Evolution, on the other hand, makes change seem like an organic moment. Vimal, while pitching his ideas for the department, should have made it seem like it was a collective plan for the department by everyone, not just by him. This way, it would have seemed like an organic evolution coming from the department and not solely from Vimal. This would have given Vimal the advantage of having created stakeholders for his ideas, rather than the opposition he faced. The same applies to your family and your relatives. Don't try to enforce changes upon them, try instead to introduce changes organically. For instance, if one of your parents has diabetes and you suddenly tell them that you are no longer going to allow any sugar in the house, your effort to improve your parent's health is likely to fail. But if you slowly try to decrease the sugar in a calibrated manner, the evolution in the habit begins and you are more likely to succeed.

Remember the workplace is not a battlefield; you don't need revolutions. Try to change things from within rather than impose change from the top.

'So, there you have it Vimal,' I said. 'The Yoga Institute's five-star method to reset your work life. Do you see what you could have done differently?' I asked.

Vimal nodded and walked nearer to the moat and the gazebo.

'Hansaji, I went about it all wrong! I should have been fired a long time ago. I really did trouble both my students and my colleagues. They have been so patient . . . no, downright considerate towards me,' he exclaimed.

'The mind, Vimal, is your most flexible tool! It is also your most rigid part,' I said, looking up at the birds chirping in the kailashpati tree near the gazebo.

Vimal nodded, 'My mind was so rigid, Hansaji. I was so caught up in one way of doing things—my way of doing things—that I completely lost track of everything else. My rigidity was completely against everything I had learned. During my research, we were always urged to value and respect opinions that were different from our own. But in the workplace, I conveniently chose to forget this.'

'Vimal, the workplace is where the real learning begins. Life is your teacher and experiences, both good and bad, are your constant companions. Whatever happens when you get back to Indore, you have learnt invaluably from your mistakes and you will be the richer for it,' I said.

Vimal stood near the edge of the gazebo, removed one chappal and then another and smiled a genuine, heart-warming smile.

'That is so true, Hansaji. If nothing, my mistakes have taught me that my mind can sometimes play tricks on me and make me think that my way is the only way. However, I have learnt that it does not need to be so.'

And slowly, the stern professor from Indore dipped one foot and then the other, into the water running around the gazebo. 'This feels light; calm. **Letting go has not been easy, but it has been worthwhile.**' He looked into the distance with the serene acceptance of all that he had learnt and all that life was yet to teach him.

The water rumbled and tumbled around our feet as **it took away from us the weary burden of our worries and brought to us the calm and connectedness of the wide world that we are all part of.**

Over the years, a lot of people have asked me whether the five-star method really works. I have never been a person to impose my views or opinions on other. **But I advise people to believe in the results they see.** This, I have always said and will say for the five-star method as well.

The bright lights of the auditorium flashed at us and a thunderous applause echoed from all corners of the auditorium. I watched as a shy but thrilled Vimal walked onto the stage and stood next to me to collect the award for several years of distinguished service and leadership. I was so happy to see my student so successful. I handed him his trophy, but he bowed and touched my feet. 'None of this would be possible without you, Hansaji. The five-star method changed my life. I am indebted to you.'

'Vimal, there is no greater joy in celebrating the success of my students. I taught you what I knew, but **it takes real courage to learn from your mistakes and try to learn something new,**' I said with a smile. Vimal accepted the trophy from me and smiled as he was cheered by his many friends and supporters.

The lights shone brighter, as though covering us all in the glow of some surreal sunlight as the joys of success and a life lived with purpose surrounded us.

FOUR

Reset Your Relationship

'A relationship is not 50-50 . . . it's 100-100. Each person has to show up fully committed.'

—Yuri Elkaim

The soft morning rays streaked through the leaves of the mango tree and gently touched my face. I savoured the warm, glowing light and my heart filled with gratitude that we lived in a land that was nourished by the sun. As I looked up, I remembered my trip to Europe during the winter months and the joy I felt at seeing the sun after spending several days under bleak, grey skies. This trip made me realize how much there is to celebrate in life, but **we waste the best part of life fearing the worst of life!** We don't make the best decisions for our life because of this very same fear.

'Namaste, Hansaji,' said Anagha. I let go of my train of thought and turned to look at the pleasant woman before me. Anagha Srinivasan was a talented and successful investment analyst who had worked with the top investment firms in the country. A few years ago, Anagha had joined the beginner's programme at The Yoga Institute to deal with her stressful work conditions. At the end of it, however, she discovered much more than stress control with us and was now one of our most popular yoga instructors. Through yoga, Anagha had not only improved her productivity at work but also found something outside it that was a source of fulfilment for her. She had a gentle smile on her lips, the sort that accentuated her beautiful features. Her olive skin glistened with beads of sweat as she arrived for our meeting immediately after her early morning class. Though her smile lingered on her lips, I could see the worry fogging her eyes, like the grey clouds I saw in European skies many years ago.

Young and successful, Anagha had recently been caught up in a maze of fear and worry. Despite her sophisticated professional reputation, accomplishments and achievements, she was a bit of an overthinker when it came to her personal life—especially her relationships. Anagha had spent over a decade establishing her career. Now, her parents were extremely worried that she would not find a suitable match for marriage and that their only child would end up being alone in life. This concern is what led them to talk to me about Anagha's reluctance to get married. They told me that she didn't like most of the suitors they managed to find for her, and they were prepared to accept a love match if that was what their daughter wanted. However, Anagha told them that she was not dating anyone either. Things had remained in limbo for a few months, until her parents managed to find a match in Shiva for her. Both Mr and Mrs Srinivasan saw the change in Anagha's eyes when both families met for the first time. They told me that they saw sparks fly instantly between the two of them. The parents sincerely hoped that their only child would find true happiness and commitment with Shiva.

Earlier, things between Anagha and Shiva seemed to have been progressing smoothly. Both were educated, ambitious, successful and seemed to share the same life goals. The parents were quite confident that it was just a matter of time before Anagha and Shiva would announce to their respective families that they were ready to get married. However, Anagha had recently announced that she wouldn't be taking things forwards with Shiva. Stumped and exasperated, Mr and Mrs Srinivasan had asked me to talk to their daughter, complaining that they could hardly extract anything except monosyllables out of her.

And that is why Anagha had come to meet me on this gentle morning as the sun had just begun to peep out of the clouds.

'Namaste, Anagha,' I replied and offered her a seat. 'Would you like some ginger tea?' I asked as I began to pour a cup for myself. She nodded and I poured a cup for her too.

She took the tea gingerly from my hands as she sat at the edge of her seat. It was easy to see that she was uncomfortable with the situation, so I decided to head straight to the heart of the matter.

'Anagha, your parents care about you. They asked me to talk to you in the hope that it could help you.'

Anagha looked at me and said, 'But Hansaji, they do not understand me. They think of marriage as an essential aspect of life. But to me, it seems like something that would restrict my freedom.'

'What about Shiva?' I asked quietly.

'He feels the same.'

'Hmmm. Does he? Or do you both actually dislike each other?'

Anagha nodded to say that they did like each other. By the look on her face, it was clear that they both had a lot of emotions for each other and liked each other a lot. She took another sip of tea, hoping that the tiny cup would hide the sea of emotions that had begun to show on her face. However, I could clearly see that she felt deeply for Shiva. And yet, this smart, educated and successful woman was choosing to turn her face away from love and emotions. I knew she needed to reset her relationship, but I couldn't help her till I had understood more of her emotions.

But before I could say anything, she interrupted me suddenly. 'Hansaji, love and relationships are different nowadays. Things are very complicated, unlike the era my parents lived in. You wouldn't understand!' A tiny tear rolled down her cheek. Eager to stick to her image of a strong businesswoman, she brushed it away impatiently and looked at me.

'Anagha, tell me, does love get software updates like your iPhone?' I asked.

She looked at me, absolutely stumped. 'What do you mean, Hansaji?'

'Well, you said that love and relationships are different nowadays. Please tell me from where I can download the updated version of human emotions.'

Anagha chuckled. Finally, something had lightened her mood. 'Hansaji, that's not what I meant, although I understand where you're coming from . . .'

'See, Anagha, humans feel love, hate, anger, joy and jealousy the same way now as they did thousands of years ago. When you say your problems are different, you create an unnecessary distinction between yourself and others. Remember, what you are feeling today, your parents felt yesterday and your children will feel tomorrow.'

'But Hansaji . . . it feels so difficult,' she gulped.

'It's difficult only when you are scared,' I said. Anagha looked unconvinced. 'Why don't both you and Shiva meet me tomorrow morning? We can see if I need an update on my emotions or if both of you need to reset your emotions,' I said, chuckling.

Anagha smiled as she nodded in agreement and walked out. I had a feeling that tomorrow would be an interesting day; I was eager to unpack what went on inside the heads of young people today. It was an amazing mystery to me how or why people chose to forego adventures of life so easily nowadays.

The next morning, I had just finished addressing the last batch of the 21-Day Better Living course. It was heartening to hear and see how visibly different the students felt within just twenty-one days of this course. Most students would love it so much that they would do the course again; some doing so five or six times in succession. As I walked out of the Dharana auditorium, I saw Anagha waiting for me outside the hall with a tall, dark man. Shiva was impeccably dressed and had all the signs of being the successful engineer that he was. The fact that he agreed to meet me with only a day's notice, at Anagha's bidding, told me that he clearly cared about what she felt. Both Anagha and Shiva didn't seem to realize that they were inadvertently holding hands. I wished they saw each other as I saw them: two people who could create their own world and learn to share each other's joys and sorrows. And yet, they were choosing to detach from each other despite their obvious connection. I sighed as they wished me.

'Namaste Hansaji,' Anagha said.

'Namaste Hansaji,' Shiva said too. I sensed a slight discomfort in him at being in the new surroundings, but he took his cues from Anagha. If it was important for her, it seemed to be important for him as well. I saw a very real concern in his eyes for her. It reminded me of how Dr Jayadev, my husband, would always keep cloves in his pocket whenever we lectured as he knew the long hours irritated my throat. These sweet memories made me grateful for all the time I got to spend with him.

I smiled at him and though he smiled back, he seemed unsure about being at the institute.

'Namaste and welcome to the Yoga Institute,' I said.

'Thank you, Hansaji. Anagha has told me a lot about this place and I know how much it means to her.'

I smiled again. 'Anagha is one of our most popular teachers. She is well-liked by the students and staff alike.'

Anagha beamed and Shiva seemed delighted to see her happy. I guided them towards my office where we could sit comfortably. I offered Shiva some of our famous ginger tea. He seemed sceptical about it since he preferred the original kind. But at Anagha's prodding, he was willing to try ginger tea and sipped it tentatively as Anagha looked on expectantly. He looked back and said, 'It's nice, Anagha.' Anagha grinned and then blushed a little as she realized that I was there.

I couldn't help myself; I saw two people, who had strong emotions for each other, continue to deny their feelings.

'Both of you feel deeply for each other,' I said, coming straight to the point. 'Shiva, you are willing to do things just to make her happy and Anagha, you seem to have an implicit trust that he will be there for you. Also, I asked him to join us with very little notice and he seems to have found the time because it mattered to you,' I said.

They both nodded at me, looked at each other and then at the floor, somehow afraid to admit to their emotions for each other. Though they were fully grown adults they looked like scared children who had been caught by the principal.

I was puzzled. 'Why do you not want to be together when you clearly care so much for each other and make each other happy?'

Shiva answered, 'Hansaji, I have had difficult experiences in my earlier relationships. They make it difficult for me to trust people with my emotions, especially in relationships. I wish I'd met Anagha during my college days before my mind was coloured by negative experiences.' He let out a deep sigh and covered his face with his hands.

'It's not just him, Hansaji,' said Anagha defensively. 'I find it difficult to say yes to marriage. I see it as something that would restrict my freedom. I am used to taking my own decisions in life and career and wouldn't like it if somebody else interfered with them.'

These statements were perfect examples of how we use our minds to create problems when there are none. Patiently, I turned to Shiva and asked, 'If you slipped on a banana peel once, would you stop eating bananas forever?'

He seemed somewhat embarrassed now. Perhaps he had begun to understand the fallacy in the assumption that every relationship would be a source of pain.

He smiled a crooked smile at himself and replied, 'Umm . . . no, Hansaji. And I know Anagha is so different from anyone I have ever met before. But I am so caught up in what happened before . . .' he trailed off.

'Falling into a ditch is a painful experience, especially if you fall several times. Nobody is denying or underplaying the difficulties you faced. But as you said yourself, it happened in the past. If you keep looking backwards, then you will always drive the car of your life in reverse gear. Learn to look ahead in life. Learn from the past but live in the present; act to create a bright future for yourself.' I added.

I then turned to face Anagha, who was nodding in complete agreement, 'You studied economics, didn't you Anagha?' I asked.

She nodded.

'Define 'profit' for me, please.'

'Profit is the reward for taking risk, Hansaji' she replied.

'In economics, if you can expect profits only after risk, then why not expect the same in your personal relationships? You have simply assumed that marriage will curtail your freedom. Have you asked yourself if it's because you are afraid of the risk?' I asked.

Anagha looked thoughtful.

'The problem begins when you see marriage simply as a set of rituals or obligations that seek to bind you. It is so much more than that. Marriage does not try to bind or restrict your freedom at all. It is an adventure that you take with someone when you wish to share life's joys and sorrows and access parts of yourself that were perhaps hidden from you too,' I added.

'Hansaji, if marriage is not simply a set of rituals, what is it?' Anagha asked.

'Marriage, in the Vedic tradition, assigns a lot of importance to *saptapadi* or the seven sacred vows. Each vow is not a mere ritual, but rather a promise that the couple makes to each other.'

1. **Strength:** The vow states, 'Let us be happy, enjoy life and grow together in strength.'
2. **Prosperity:** The vow states, 'Let us walk together so that we get wealth, trust each other and be loyal.'
3. **Friendship:** The vow states, 'Let us be friends and share in all our joys and sorrows. Let us find a home in each other as friends.'
4. **Intimacy:** The vow states, 'Let us find love with each other and open ourself to being open and intimate with each other.
5. **Discover your emotions:** The vow states, 'In this step of married life, let us discover our emotions for each other and for ourself.
6. **Ego:** The vow states, 'Let us live peacefully without any clashes of ego in our life.
7. **Family:** The vow states, 'Let us promise to care for each other's families. Let our marriage bear witness to the joys of family life and loving care.'

'But Hansaji, these seem like theoretical ideas,' argued Shiva. 'Are these relevant to relationships today?'

'Shiva, something remains theoretical when we fail to practice it in real life. Trust and commitment in relationships remains theoretical when we are not loyal to our partners. Unconditional love remains theoretical when we base it on conditions like wealth or social status,' I said.

'Hansaji is right, Shiva. We see many couples who attend couples' counselling workshops at the institute. I have seen how many of their problems crop up from within themselves; from their own insecurities or irrational expectations,' said Anagha.

I looked at Shiva, who still looked sceptical. Doubt, I have always believed, is at the root of almost all our problems. So, I decided to show Shiva how relevant the 'mere rituals' (as he called it) were to marriage and any relationship in general.

'Shiva, when we consciously decide to practice what you think of as theoretical rituals; our marriages, our lives and relationships bloom from within. Each vow becomes the guiding force of a fulfilling and happy relationship. And you will see how they work to make your relationship better. Let's go over some examples.'

Seven Steps to Successful Relationships

1. Learning acceptance or walking together to grow in strength

Karan and Anusha met in college and married after a few years of courtship. In time, they realized that while loving each other is one thing, living with each other is a whole different ballgame. They had differences. Karan needed everything to be ordered and organized; Anusha liked going with the flow. Karan had impeccable to-do lists for the day and monthly and yearly plans for his life. Anusha, on the other hand, liked not knowing; she enjoyed surprises. When they'd dated, these habits had seemed like cute idiosyncrasies, but living together, they had become irritants. The two tried to overlook these as mere differences of temperament. But the more they swept them under the carpet, the starker these differences became.

Karan and Anusha had been brought up in completely different households. Born into a military family, Karan had always valued discipline, order and organization. Anusha's parents, on the other hand, had been artists who believed in ease, comfort and artistic liberties. They were different but marriage is always supposed to be a union of different halves. What one misses, the other provides; that's how two halves become whole. Both Karan and Anusha had so much to learn from each other. But learning only comes from a place of acceptance; acceptance that you can love people who are different from you. Love is not dependent on conditions of similarity. If conditions are imposed, then one is coming from a place of ego, not love. The ego likes control and more than control, it likes to live with what is comfortable. It views anything different as a threat to its presence. With ego, marriage becomes a game of control; with love, marriage becomes a game of cards. In this game, you must accept the cards that have been dealt to you and play the best possible game you can with them. Remember, you don't throw away your cards because you think you have a bad hand. At the end of a Hindu wedding, there is a ceremony called *dhruva darshan* where the priest asks the newlyweds to gaze at the *dhruva nakshatra* or the polestar together. This ritual symbolizes a shift in perspective as the newlyweds begin the journey of the marriage together. They do not view the polestar separately but as a united couple. This does not mean that either party has compromised their viewpoints, it simply means that they have begun to share perspectives. Gradually, they evolve their own unique perspective; a new way of seeing the world. *Dhruva darshan* symbolizes the steadfastness of their bond despite the challenges of the universe.

What happened with Karan and Anusha was that they were too caught up in their own ways to appreciate what they had to offer to one another. Though Anusha understood the benefits of organization and order, she thought that accepting it would mean that she was *giving in* to Karan. And Karan thought being a little more relaxed about things would imply that Anusha was right and that his upbringing and values were faulty. Each saw the other's viewpoint as a threat to their identity, which is inadvisable. It should instead be seen as a chance to explore new ideas and experiences that we would not have had if we were on our own. No two people can ever be completely alike. Some qualities will be in sync and others will be different. Besides, if two people are the same, there will be nothing to learn, nothing to talk about and nothing to discover.

When Karan and Anusha came to me, I knew it was a question of perspective for them. I decided to counsel them using an exercise that I now call 'dhruva darshan' after the ritual whose meaning and significance we forget so often. I had a box that changed colour when it was placed in the darkness. It was blue in the light and when the light was switched off, it turned red. I sent Karan and Anusha to check the colour of the box, one after the other.

'What was the colour of the box?' I asked when both returned.

'Blue,' said Karan.

'Red,' said Anusha.

'You always want to contradict me, Anusha,' grumbled Karan.

'Well, you never agree with anything I do,' retorted Anusha.

They started arguing and I could sense the strain such constant and acrimonious disagreements would have on their marriage. If they continued like this, their marriage would soon fall apart or lose any real affection and concern. It was high time that they reset their emotions to reset their marriage. I asked Rohita to get the box from the other room so that the matter could be settled then and there. She entered the room with the box in her hands and Karan had a smile that stretched from ear to ear as he saw the blue box. Anusha looked completely stumped.

'I told you, Anusha!' he exclaimed, 'You never believe me.'

'But . . . but . . . it was red, Hansaji!' insisted Anusha.

'Rohita, switch the lights off,' I said.

Rohita switched off the lights and the box turned red.

'Yes!' shrieked Anusha. It was Karan's turn to look stumped and my turn to make them see some sense before their marriage fell apart.

Rohita switched the lights on again and the box turned blue.

'You are both so obsessed with what you think is right that you don't even bother about your partner's perspective.

Neither one of you had the sense or concern to listen or talk to your partner about what they saw. The only thing that mattered to you was being right,' I said.

They both looked down to the floor like little children who had been caught having a silly fight.

'When you want to be right in your marriage all the time, the marriage goes wrong in no time.' They both looked at each other and then at me. It looked like some of what I had said had begun to make sense to them. Slowly, they moved towards each other and held hands.

'I should have asked,' said Karan.

'I should have listened,' said Anusha.

'Yes, you should have,' I said. 'See, marriage is like this box. Sometimes it's blue, other times it's red. At times, you may see it as one colour and your partner may see it as another. But that doesn't mean you turn against one another just because you don't see the same colour.'

They nodded.

'Remember, when you both got married you must have probably performed the *dhruvadarshan* ritual where you both viewed the pole star together. That was not mere ritual, it was meant to teach you the value of seeing things together; accepting each other's perspective.'

They both looked at me with understanding.

'Anusha, I was so determined to be right that I couldn't see how things affected you,' Karan said.

'I too was hell-bent on setting you straight, Karan,' Anusha said.

'If you expect your partner to be exactly like you, then you should have married yourself. When you are with someone else, you both must learn to share your lives with one another. If things don't always match; if your partner has what you consider defects, remember they are not something you bought from an online store that you can return! And you definitely can't get a refund on your marriage!' I said.

This got a laugh from them as they walked happily out of the room together. Rohita and I smiled at each other.

> Remember in marriage, it's about accepting them as they are and not expecting them to be as you are.

2. Managing finances or prosperity

Marriage is never about one person being completely responsible for anything. It is about finding a supportive partner for everything. It is never a one-way street in anything, not even finances. Though you are free to choose whether you want to work or not, irrespective of gender, you are not free of the financial responsibilities of the partnership. Before you get married, discussing concerns like retirement plans, investment goals and financial aims is vital. Most marriages run into trouble when partners have different financial goals and aspirations. If you are okay with a one-room apartment but your partner has always desired a villa, your marriage will soon crumble. It's like one wheel of an engine wants to go towards the west and the other wheel wants to travel to the east. Just imagine what kind of journey would that be?

This was exactly the case with Parmanu and Aishwarya. Parmanu was born with a silver spoon in his mouth and believed in living expansively. Born into affluence and having all his needs met unconditionally, Parmanu wasn't keen on saving or investing his wealth. He believed that he would always have access to more than enough wealth to finance his lavish lifestyle. Aishwarya, meanwhile, was born into an ordinary family and understood the value and importance of money. She also knew how easily you could lose money if it was not used wisely. Aishwarya's frugal and mature approach to money was one of the key reasons why Parmanu's parents chose her as their son's bride. They had hoped that Aishwarya's frugality would strike a balance against Parmanu's extravagance. However, the marriage was rocky because neither had made the effort to discuss finances at all. This led to Parmanu resenting Aishwarya's approach, which he considered stingy. Meanwhile, Aishwarya thought that Parmanu blatantly disrespected money.

Things came to a head because they couldn't resolve this fundamental difference in their beliefs. They would have certainly divorced had a case of bad luck not struck Parmanu's business. Faced with mounting losses and decreasing incomes, Parmanu began to value Aishwarya and her approach to handling money and Aishwarya began to appreciate the hard work Parmanu put in to set things straight in business. She found cause to respect him, which became a strong enough reason for love to bloom in her heart. With some help from the couples' workshop at the institute, they dropped the idea of divorce and also laid the foundation of a solid relationship based on mutual respect. Adversity turned out to be lucky for Parmanu and Aishwarya. But most of us are not so lucky and what begins as small disagreements about money, soon becomes why people line up outside the family court for divorce.

Be practical and realize that without money, there can be no success in life or marriage. Find someone who shares your financial values and goals. If not, at least be with someone who can respect what you stand for. If you think that after marriage you will manage to convince someone of your viewpoint or that they will have no choice but to agree to the way you do things, you both are bound to be miserable. Spare yourself the tears and talk to your partner regarding money woes and wishes!

3. Cultivating friendship in marriage

In Mahabharata, Yaksha asks Yudhisthira, *'Kimsvin mitram grihesatah?'* Who is the friend of the householder? Yudhisthira replies, 'The friend of the householder is their spouse.' When a newly married couple takes the vow of friendship during the saptapadi, they say, 'With these seven steps, you have become my friend. May I deserve your friendship. May my friendship make me one with you. May your friendship make you one with me.'

Marriage needs friendship. If a couple is together for twenty years, they spend an average of 7300 days (or 1,75,200 hours) in each other's company. This is more than enough time to melt a tonne of ice in Antarctica. If that much time can do that to the ice in Antarctica, imagine what that will do to you. If you do not spend that time with a friend, with someone that loves and cares for you, you would also melt from the inside.

Most of us falter when we think that there is no effort required to build a friendship within the marriage. It is very easy to get irritated by the fact that we aren't getting time to ourselves, but it is a different game altogether when we try to be a little more sensitive to our partner's needs. In marriage or relationships, making an effort for the other person doesn't make you weak or small. It simply means that you are mature enough to understand the importance of making an effort for another person. But make sure it's not a one-way street. You should also receive the same amount of attention and care from the other person. This mutuality is the true essence of friendship in any relationship.

When there is a sense of friendship in a marriage, there is an unsaid understanding that there is acceptance and trust in the marriage. This is because you don't have expectations that your friend has to be so rich or successful. Generally, we are friends with people because we believe that they will accept us for who we are without judgment. If we can do that for our friends, then why can we not do that for our partners or spouses? Once we are friends with them, the comfort levels in the relationship go through the roof and it is a recipe for assured success.

There are umpteen benefits of being friends with your partner or spouse. You **get to have a lot of fun with each other.** You'll have **a partner in crime for all your adventures**. And finally, **you'll never be alone. You'll always have someone to care for and someone who cares for you.**

4.   Developing love and intimacy

But love is not just about being friends. What makes relationships born out of love one of the most satisfying, profound and mysterious human experiences is how there are so many layers to it. **You can never fully understand it but you can always fully experience it**. Friendship is an important part of love but not its only part. There are elements of intimacy which are both emotional and sexual. In the time of Tinder, one would expect a sexual revolution to be taking place. However, the ease of being able to have sex has done nothing to help people accept their sexuality. Instead, it has put an added element of pressure in terms of accessing their sexual identities. Sexual intimacy comes from a place of caring for your partner's needs and satisfaction. But the modern dating industry is constructed on the basis of instant pleasure; a principle designed to make you focus only on yourself. Developing intimacy requires a degree of commitment. That is why your flings leave you feeling unsatisfied and inadequate after the initial rush. The absence of intimacy, comfort and trust in your relationships with people makes you question whether you are worthy of love or not, one of the most natural questions we often always ask ourselves. If the answer is more often a 'no', it can hurt our sense of self greatly. Therefore, before you embark on your next fling, ask yourself if it's just about having fun or if it's about avoiding making yourself vulnerable to real human emotions and feelings. If it's a yes to the latter, it is time for you to reset your emotions around sex, love and intimacy.

Remember true intimacy comes only from a place of acceptance of yourself. You have to take the step to accept and love yourself only then can you, provide for the emotional needs of others. This acceptance of yourself nurtures a sense of intimacy within you, for you. And once you learn the definition of intimacy like this you learn to apply it with others as well. So, through this emotional rebalancing within you find the space and the capacity for true physical intimacy with your partner. True physical intimacy means that it is something that you actively desire. It comes from a place of love and acceptance of yourself, your partner and your relationship. So don't rush into anything if you are not comfortable about. Many women and sometimes even men, think they are obligated to give in sexually just because they are married or in a relationship with someone. Remember you are never obligated to do anything you are uncomfortable with. Always talk to your partner about what is okay for you and what is not. This serves many functions. First, it establishes better communication in the relationship. Second, it implies to your partner that you trust them enough to tell them of your needs. In a true relationship, no partner would disregard what you need. If you see your partner belittling your concerns it's time to take a tough, realistic look at how healthy your relationship really is.

See relationships are not about two halves coming together to make a full. Instead they are about two complete people choosing to create a new life together. An intimate, healthy and happy relationship is not possible when two halves come together because in such a case both parties simply want to take and not give. Often people lie to themselves that they are in love when in fact they are simply going through the motions of a need-based relationship. If you are in a relationship to heal a wound, then it's simply a need-based relationship. The important question you need to ask yourself is **'Am I in love or am I in need?'** An emotionally centered person always has the confidence to give and care for their partners than someone who comes from a space of need. Therefore, reset your emotions to come from a place of care and commitment and see how soon you will invite intimacy and satisfaction into your life.

5.   Discovering your emotions.

In marriage, understanding is only possible if we understand our own emotions first. Most of our challenges develop when we do not understand them. For instance, we often think we are angry, but as one poet said, behind anger, there is always grief. And behind grief, there is always love which has nowhere to go. The anger you feel for your spouse is often caused by the idea that they hurt you in some way. The anger is a mask for the grief.

Let's visit another case. Sumitra and Nitin had been engaged for three months and were preparing for their big day with great fanfare. Since Sumitra was a trained singer, Nitin had requested that she record a song for him. Though talented, Sumitra never thought she was good enough and so, while sending Nitin a recording of her song, she told him, quite clearly, to not share it with anyone else. She thought this version of the song did not do her talent justice. But soon she realized that Nitin had let his office colleagues listen to her sing. Infuriated, Sumitra got into a huge row with Nitin three days before their wedding. Behind Sumitra's anger was grief. Her grief came from the belief that she was not good enough at singing. She was angry because she thought Nitin was blind to her feelings and ignored the fact that Nitin did not try to hide her from his colleagues. When your partner doesn't hide you from the world, it is a sign of commitment. In her anger, Sumitra didn't realize that and insisted that Nitin change the way he expressed his emotions or showed care. People try to change their partners because most of us know that changing the self is a daunting task. But a successful relationship develops only when we are self-assured and confident. Marriage and/or relationships help us see beyond ourselves, expand our horizons and become less self-centred. However, this can happen only when we can learn to question our emotions and learn to identify their causes instead of acting on them in haste.

6. Conquering Ego

The Yoga Sutra identifies five main kleshas or obstacles to happiness that cloud your mind. These are avidya (ignorance), asmita (over-identifying with your ego), raga (excess desire), dvesha (avoidance) and abhinivesha (attachment or fear. The ego is a hinderance to everything in most if not all philosophies. The Sanskrit word for the ego or '*Ahamkara*' derives from the root words '*aham*' or self and '*kara*' or created thing.

Archana and Devashish had met while working at one of the Big Four companies. Both had very promising careers and they were thrilled to have found someone who shared and understood so much of their work. They were soon married and things went on smoothly for some time. But soon Devashish began to have a few setbacks at work. Meanwhile Archana was offered a position to lead an international project. The generally understanding and supportive Devashish couldn't digest this, perhaps because his own career was not flourishing. The ego reared its ugly head and Devashish began to see Archana's success as a threat to his own identity. Jealousy is one of the most common ways in which the ego manifests itself in our life. Gradually their fights became a daily affair and that's how they ended up at the Couple's Workshop at The Yoga Institute.

At these sessions we routinely see how most relationships are destroyed when the ego comes into play. This imbalanced ego rears its head in many ways: trying to be right, shutting your partner out, comparison, possessiveness, making unfair demands from your partner, etc.

When the ego is over-active it puts our emotions in an unbalanced state. Insecure emotions make people defensive and so they want **to be right always.** We think it makes us small if we are wrong! Often, the need to be right is coming from your own insecurity. So if you try to be right all the time, your relationship will be wrong very soon in no time!

Remember, love is not wrong or right.
But in love, the heart is strong and bright.

The next ego-related error that can ruin your relationship is **shutting your partner out.** If your partner made a mistake or you're facing any problems, you may begin to ignore them and avoid them. Doing so, you're shutting them out. If you don't tell them about your problems then you are shutting them out. This makes them feel de-valued and that they do not matter to you. This is how distance creeps into the strongest

of relationships. Remember no relationship can survive
without communication. So no matter how bad things may
seem always be mindful that you need to give time, space and
acceptance to your partners.

Comparison is another way the ego tries to assert
dominance and control. Do you compare your partner with
your ex? Do you compare your partner with the partners of
your siblings, cousins or friends? See when you go to buy
vegetables do you see the vegetable seller weigh one kg of
tomatoes and one kg of potatoes together? No right? Then
why do you put different people in the same scale?

> Understand this: When you compare, they think you don't care.
> It is when you care unconditionally that you repair!

Another common ego problem is over-possessiveness. The
problem starts when one partner expects the other to **only
be their person and nothing else.** Over-possessive may
look like asking you to not meet friends of the opposite
gender or being annoyed when you plan to spend time
with your friends or have to spend extra hours at work or
asking you to change what you are wearing. See, understand
this that no relationship can survive this! So before over-
possessiveness ruins your relationship take concrete steps
to save it. **Understand that the first and foremost need of
any relationship is freedom. You need to feel free and not
caged in the relationship.** If you constantly impose checks
and restrictions on them, they will hardly enjoying being
with you. If you feel that your partner's over-possessiveness

is caging you in: it's time to talk thing out in the open with them. Understand that their over-possessiveness stems from the deep-rooted insecurity of the Ego. **Talk to them gently and firmly about the need to address this insecurity and create healthier boundaries in the relationship**. State firmly that you are in this relationship as an equal partner and not a kid looking for constant direction and correction on what you can or cannot do.

> Remember your most important relationship is the one you have with yourself. Don't lose yourself for the sake of being with another person.

The ego also creates demanding partners. How do you deal with demanding partners? Do you feel like you're the ATM in your relationship? Do you feel drained and exhausted by the constant demands that are set before you? Our relationships are meant to be the source of our strength; our strongest anchor here in this world. If we feel drained by what should make us powerful, then we are clearly doing something wrong.

Where does it go wrong then? We falter when we see our relationships as simple transactions where demands are made by one party and fulfilled by another. But if this is what it has become, try this.

Firstly, ask yourself if making and fulfilling demands is how love and affection is measured in your relationship. Have you unknowingly drifted away to a place where one partner believes that the other loves them only if they fulfil their needs? If so, begin by committing your time to each other again. As you choose to spend more time, you will realize that the boundaries of your love are quite beyond demand and supply. Generally, partners become demanding when they feel insignificant, unseen, or unheard in relationships and behave like children who throw tantrums when they want their parent's attention. **Re-commit your time and appreciation to your partner and see how little they will come to need from you.**

Secondly, do you feel that even after this there might be demands that would feel excessive to you? Talk to your partner. Discuss why their demands are important for them and plan together on how you can work towards them. Discuss how much time you would need to achieve this and what sacrifices would you have to make as a family to get there. **Do it together and trust me, whether you fulfil their demand or not, you will definitely have strengthened your bond.**

Relationships are not mechanical ATMs where you punch in your demand and get what you want. But when you work together as a team, demands turn into shared life goals and you realize that relationships are blank cheques of love and trust that you write out to each other. So, smile that someone wrote you a blank cheque in love. What else can you demand? Remember to hold and cherish each other till death do you part.

In the *Bhagavat Gita*, Lord Krishna explains to Arjuna the need to remove *ahamkara*. The *Gita* suggests that with *ahamkara*, the true self can never exist. The same is valid for relationships and emotions. With *ahamkara* in the centre, you will never be able to gauge the needs of your partner or relationships. Most of your emotions will be geared up to satisfy the 'I' of the *ahamkara*. Reset your emotions by leaving the *ahamkara* behind and you will see the entire world open for you.

7. Family

Vikul and Surbhi had been married for a couple of years. They were used to a set way of life and certain routines. But when Surbhi's mother had an unexpected cardiac attack, the couple was faced with a dilemma. Should they hire someone to care for Surbhi's mother or bring her to their house and look after her? They felt guilty about leaving her alone with an unknown healthcare professional and eventually, they convinced her to join them in Mumbai. Though their decision was made out of kindness and consideration, they had to make significant adjustments and changes to their lifestyles so that Surbhi's mother would feel comfortable. Vikul, aware of his duties as a son-in-law, a responsible husband and a caring friend of Surbhi, more than welcomed the decision. Surbhi's mother made a slow recovery and it took a considerable toll on the couple's time and efforts. Surprisingly, however, they found that going through something difficult brought them much closer to each other. They were more attuned to each other's thoughts, moods and needs than before. The care that they provided Surbhi's mother nourished their marital bond with love. This is the essence of the vow of family. Marriage, in the traditional sense of the term, is a union of families that connects us to people, their memories and their legacies. It is through this connectedness that we grow. We grow when we can grow with others. We grow when we find in our hearts the capacity to love and care for others.

In another instance, Shehnaaz was engaged to marry Amir in an extravagant ceremony soon. After their marriage, Shehnaaz agreed to shift from Lucknow to Hyderabad, where Amir's family was based. But as the wedding drew closer, Shehnaaz began to resent that she had to move to another city. She couldn't appreciate the efforts Amir's family were putting in to make sure their new daughter-in-law felt welcome. Amir's parents had remodelled an entire wing just for her. Yet, Shehnaaz rued over the fact that she would never find another family like her own and that she would have to make major adjustments. Relationships are never about stasis. They are challenges that push you forwards in life. If Shehnaaz had not been blinded by her attachment to her family, she might have seen the love Amir's family had for a person they had come to know recently. Relationships need you to be open to newer ideas of family and bonding. Adapting and accepting the expansions of our boundaries makes us realize that love comes in all shapes and sizes.

Many times, we hear stories of how parents have been abandoned or moved to old-age homes when married children find it difficult to care for them. People have started to believe that family puts extra strain on their marital relationships. Sometimes, there is too much of a difference in the perspective of family members. In these situations, distance goes a long way in building better relationships. But this doesn't always have to be so. Most of the time, our parents, elders and family members can be a source of strength and support for us. When we are with them, we receive support when tackling life's challenges. Marriage, in the traditional sense, makes us appreciative of this because you did not simply marry the person you married an entire family. So in your marriage and in your heart always try to find space for your spouse's family and relations. This will only work to strengthen your relationship by leaps and bounds.

> Remember, it is easy to break a single stick. But when a single stick is with a bundle of sticks, it is as strong as the entire bundle.

'So, Shiva, Anagha. What do you think?' I asked.

'Hansaji, we are already the best of friends,' said Shiva.

'And the acceptance and trust we have for each other is not ordinary. I have never felt like this before,' said Anagha.

'Yes, and you've cleared up many of the misconceptions I had about getting married, Hansaji,' added Shiva.

'You two were simply scared. Nowadays, you assume that being unattached or unmarried is a sign of freedom. The truth is that, more often than not, it is simply a comfort zone within which you have become used to doing things in certain ways. With the right person, any relationship becomes an unlimited source of freedom because you have support and companionship,' I said, as we all walked out of my office.

It was now dusk. The stars had begun to twinkle in the inky-black night sky. But one stood fixed, unwavering, despite the great distance that separated us: the *dhruvanakshatra* or the pole star.

'Hansaji, look, it's the dhruvanakshatra,' Anagha said.

I moved forwards and placed Shiva's hand in Anagha's hand and as they both looked at me, surprised, I said, 'Look at the dhruvanakshatra together, Shiva, Anagha. By doing so, let today be the beginning of a shift in your perspectives. From today, honour your relationship with the gift of a shared worldview. From today, honour the fact that you have agreed to share your lives with each other. Be excited about the fact that you have someone now to share yourself and your world with. Gradually, you evolve a new ideal of seeing and being in the world that belongs to both of you. Let today's *dhruvadarshan* reset your emotions and help you accept the profoundness of your relationship with all its joys and its unlimited potential,' I said.

With my words, I saw two young hearts look up at the *dhruvanaksahtra* with all the love they had for each other. The power of their relationship evoked a silent and powerful blessing in my heart for them. I was grateful that I could help them reset their relationship and that I could help them accept their love for each other in the truest sense.

FIVE A

Seven Golden Rules for Good Sleep

'Sleep helps you win at life.'

—Amy Poehler

Till now, we have gone over how we can reset our work life, our social life, our perspectives and our emotions. It is vital that we are balanced in these areas so that we can have meaningful and satisfying lives. However, none of this is possible till we become conscious of three things: sleep, exercise and food. These three aspects are the foundations of healthy living and well-being. Yet, these three are also the most overlooked. Looking after sleep, diet and exercise requires simple efforts from our end. However, just because the efforts are simple doesn't mean the results are not powerful.

Resetting anything in our life is impossible if we do consider food, exercise and sleep. For instance, if we are unwell, our food has the capacity to become medicine and heal us. What we put in our bodies is what shows up on our bodies. So if you choose to eat fat and sugar rich food, it will show up as layers of flab on your body. Similarly, exercise has the potential to do wonders for our body, not just physically, but emotionally and mentally as well. And any doubt about the importance of sleep as a biological function and as the basis of mental and physical health is misplaced. Sleep is vital for any creature to function. It is this understanding that perhaps compelled regimes through the centuries to use sleep deprivation as a method of torture. Depriving anyone of their rest is tantamount to inflicting the cruellest form of torment upon them.

There is an interesting anecdote that attests to the importance of sleep in a person's life. It is said that years ago, an old tyrant invited guests to a medieval palace in the heart of his kingdom. This secret palace, it was believed, was filled with every conceivable luxury. The guests were presented with an array of rich, delightful food and drink. Anything they wanted or needed would be arranged for them. There was no bar on the luxuries they could enjoy. But the tyrant had one condition for his guests: they could not sleep in his palace, not even for a minute.

What Happened Then?

The guests went through excruciating torture without sleep. They were fatigued, some began hallucinating and others were soon on their way to completely losing their minds. They had everything a person would need to live an uber-luxurious life. But without sleep none of these luxuries meant anything. This anecdote demonstrates how important sleep is for us. And yet, we often choose to sacrifice it! So, I will introduce you to the seven golden rules for good sleep. These rules are relevant for persons of any age and they will doubtless transform all areas of your life for the better.

But before that let's take a quick look at what exactly sleep does for us.

A 2020 study on sleep patterns in India found that one in four Indians felt that they have a sleep disorder. Those living in metropolitan cities had the worst sleep quality and 80 per cent of youth under the age of eighteen admitted that they felt tired after waking up. Another 50 per cent of teenagers under eighteen also felt that they have insomnia.

Our frenzied, competitive lives today have ensured that we have a twenty-four-hour supply of stress and endless work. All this has thrown our sleep cycles for a toss. Our numerous entertainment choices in television or streaming services or social media have further exacerbated this situation. Misplaced priorities of earning more and more coupled with a general idea that sleep is a symbol of laziness and lethargy has done great, irreparable harm to many of us. Many adults and children preparing for competitive exams supposedly sleep for less than five hours a day. Studies show that low sleep increases mortality causes by more than 15 per cent.

Sleep is important for every part and process of the body and mind. While it may seem like the body is doing nothing, getting good rest is important for our immunity, mental health, cognitive functioning and metabolism. While we sleep, the body performs vital repair tasks such as protein synthesis at a cellular level, among other important functions.

Sleep helps us with weight loss. It does! If you have been trying to lose weight and failing, look at your sleep patterns. What happens is at night, when we sleep soundly, we tend to burn more calories. Neurotransmitters such as ghrelin and leptin control hunger and satiation in our bodies. Ghrelin causes feelings of hunger in us while leptin causes the feeling of satiety after meals. A lack of sleep may affect the body's ability to regulate these neurotransmitters. For instance, if your body keeps producing ghrelin and lesser amounts of leptin, you could end up constantly feeling hunger, leading to increased food intake and that would adversely affect any weight loss plans a person might have. Studies also suggest that sleep-deprived people prefer food that is high in calories and carbohydrates, which might be challenging for folks. Extra time spent being awake may also increase opportunities to eat, disturbing the body's natural circadian rhythms, leading to additional weight gain.

Good sleep makes you more productive and creative throughout the day. Sleeping and waking up at the same time helps maintain the natural circadian rhythms of the human body. An imbalance between daily routines and the body's internal clock can act as a trigger for lifestyle diseases, alter a person's sleeping habits, cause mood changes and affect their emotional health.

Sleep also has a metaphysical aspect. While you sleep, it is believed that you enter an altered state of consciousness. In this state, you are free from the limits of your minds, identities and burdens. This allows you to connect with and access the limitlessness of the universal consciousness. Metaphysicists believe this is vital to the process of physical, emotional and mental regeneration, healing and cleansing.

Now that we know how much good sleep can help us, let's go over **the seven golden rules for good sleep.**

1. **Sleep not with a full belly but with a happy belly:** The first golden rule of good sleep is regarding the vital secret of how to keep the belly happy. The key to this is simple: keep a gap of two to three hours between dinner and bedtime.

   Dinner is the last meal of the day and should always be light to avoid health problems. The logic behind eating a light dinner at least two hours before bedtime is very simple—it gives the body enough time to digest the food. For instance, when you eat a large meal right before bedtime, you are putting extra stress on your digestive system to work overtime in order to process all the food you have put into it! By evening, the metabolism of the body slows down and so do biological processes such as digestion. The food eaten needs more time to get digested than it would in the day. When there is a suitable gap between dinner and bedtime, the body gets the necessary time to digest dinner completely.

   If you eat a heavy meal close to bedtime, your digestion slows down and your body uses up extra energy to digest your food. How will it find the energy for all the work it has to do while you sleep? Just imagine the amount of extra stress it puts on the body. And if you keep making your belly work overtime continuously, it will become unhappy very soon. And an unhappy belly is the fastest path to a range of diseases like acidity, bloating, weak lungs and even heart ailments.

   Why do that to yourself? Remember: happy belly, happy life!

2. **Create a happy place inside your mind:** As we discussed in earlier chapters, develop a daily habit of writing down ten positive things that happened to you during the day.

   This could be something as simple as buying a cup of tea for someone who needed it or making a note of how much you love your new shoes. Anything that touched your heart or made you feel good about yourself makes its way into the book before bedtime. This way, before you go to sleep, you will be in a happy place, which will help you sleep better. This is not simply some random concept but a very practical one too.

   When you create a happy place inside your head, your body releases all happy hormones (such as endorphins!) but when you are full of stress, the body releases cortisol, i.e., the stress hormone, which strains your heart and other vitals. It's challenging to sleep peacefully when bad hormones are raging throughout your system, especially when we all know by now how vital sleep is for us.

   So, happy to bed may not make you wealthy, but it will make you healthy and wise.

3. **Reflection:** This third golden rule is a simple, yet profound, yogic technique that inculcates *anitya bhavana* or the feeling of impermanence within us. What does that mean? Simply that it means it's a technique that helps the mind realize that all our stress and worries are impermanent. We need not carry their burdens to bed; we can sleep in peace. How do we do this? As you lie down, think of what happened in the morning, then afternoon

and then evening. Just simply think of a series of events without getting emotionally invested.

After doing so, reflect on how what happened in the morning, changed into the afternoon and how the events of the afternoon, shifted into the evening. If it helps, you can also chant the following: 'What was there in the morning that was not there in the afternoon? What was there in the afternoon that was not there in the evening? What was there in the evening that was not there in the night?'

As you say these words to yourself, you will realize how temporary your problems are and how easily you can let go of them and lapse into sleep

Remember, worry will only hurry you to your end. Why worry when you can be merry?

4. **Keep in mind the story of the goose that laid golden eggs:** What if I were to give you such a goose—what would you do? Would you be like the farmer who killed the goose or would you take care of the goose all your life? I don't know about you but I, for one, would not kill the goose that lays the golden eggs. What say? Should I give you all the magic goose? The thing is, we never realize the value of the things we have. If I told you, you all already have the golden goose, none of you would believe me. Here is the secret: our body is a golden goose. Everything you do, everything you can achieve is because of your body. Tell me one thing you can do without a healthy body.

Our next golden rule goes over how to care for the golden goose when preparing for bed every night. Before going to bed, remove all the strains and stresses of the day from the body. There are a few simple stretches that can help you do just that.

Firstly, sit on the bed and interlace your fingers. Raise both your hands above your shoulders and stretch upwards.

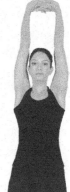

Next, lie down and raise your legs up and down, one after another. Do this for as long as it's comfortable. Once you are done, slowly lower your legs.

Finally, as you lie in bed, bend both your knees. Try to get your feet as close as you can to your hips.

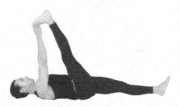

After these stretches use the Yogendra Pranayama number 4 technique to help you relax before sleeping. *Yogendra pranayama* number 4 is specifically meant to relax your nervous system. Here's how you begin:

Turn off your phone and the lights, get into comfortable clothing and lie down on your back with your feet spread apart. Bend your knees till your feet touch your hips. Keep one hand on your abdomen and the other by your side. Inhale gently and feel the belly move upward

and outward. Exhale
and feel the belly sink.
Try to inhale and exhale
for approximately the
same duration. Practice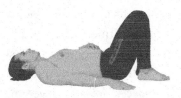
for as long as you can. Remember, you don't need to retain
or suspend your breath while you are doing this. There
should be no exaggerated movement of your abdomen.
Your breath should be slow and calm.

This rhythmic inhalation and exhalation will increase
the supply of oxygen and nutrients to every cell of your
body. This reduces the harmful effects of the stress
hormone cortisol in your body directly signalling to your
brain that it is ok to rest and relax.

A good night's sleep is mainly what affects our energy
and productivity levels the next day. People often struggle
with insomnia or sleep disorders, which are linked to
disruptions in the parasympathetic nervous system—a
system that is adversely affected by stress and anxiety. If
you want better sleep, you need to address the root cause
of your stress. Breathing techniques such as *pranayamas*
are useful for this.

5. **Sleep Sesame (So ja sim sim):** Remember the story of
Ali Baba and the forty thieves and the fantastic events
that unfolded in his life after he found the magic cave
full of untold riches? Your sleep is your source of untold
riches. To get there, you must make a magic cave for
yourself and you don't have to trek through the sands
of Arabia to get there. The magic cave is something you

create inside your bedroom by inculcating a soothing, calm atmosphere.

So every night say 'sleep sesame' and switch off the lights to have a comfortable, uninterrupted sleep in a clean space. Nowadays everything from eating to watching TV to talking is done in bed. This confuses the mind as it struggles to perceive the bed as a place of rest after a day of activity on and around it. The anxiety and frustration that you felt throughout the day remains in the bed with you when you try to sleep. So, to help your mind relax, try to make sure that your bed is exclusively a space for rest and rejuvenation. Keep it clean, do not clutter with washed clothes, unread books, or other paraphernalia. Maintain it as a sacred space where you honour your body's need for rest. Make it as comfortable as you need it to be with pillows and blankets of your choice. As you do all this, you signal to your mind that it is in a safe space where it can relax. This also suggests that you can be comfortable within your body now.

Another contrarian practice to a night of good, restful sleep is having the lights switched on. If you have the lights on, even if it's a night lamp, or the curtains are kept open, it signals your brain to remain active and respond to light stimuli. This can happen even when you get up in the middle of the night for a bathroom break. As you try to fall asleep again, light stimuli can keep your mind active. Try to make yourself comfortable in a dark room. If you are prone to anxiety attacks and feel that the darkness triggers your anxiety, reduce the intensity of light over a gradual period of time and opt for night lamps with a soft, warm and soothing glow. This subconsciously signals to the brain that it is time to sleep since it is in a space exclusively reserved for rest. There is no other activity it is expected to be performed here. As you make this a part of your daily routine, the brain will automatically begin to view the space as one meant for rest, making it possible to have an uninterrupted night of peace.

6. **Make a mental shield or a 'mind fence':** The next golden rule is a fun, creative and imaginative one. When you are on your bed, it is important to give yourself a mental break since your mind has been filled with stress and anxiety, which makes your brain overactive. At night, it is of utmost importance to give your brain a break from such chronic over-thinking so that you create space for it to rest, refresh and rejuvenate.

   The mental shield or the 'mind fence' technique is an easy and effective way to help your mind unwind and relax. You have to do the following: as you lie down on your bed, visualize an imaginary fence around your bed. Imagine that this fence has the magnetic power to extract elements such as work stress, anxiety, negative thoughts or household responsibilities from your mind. Imagine that once the fence extracts these, it keeps all these outside the fence, away from you, your body and mind.

   Next, imagine the fence creating a shield of calmness around you. Feel the lightness in your body as you let go of all these burdens you were carrying. The only things that can seep through this fence are feelings of calmness, happiness and well-being. Note it is not thoughts but simple feelings that can enter and only good feelings. Feel how light and content you are. As you lie down, imagine yourself surrounded by this fence and that it is a safe, carefree space where it is okay to let go and relax. As you feel relaxed, calm, safe and protected see sleep gently come into your eyes. Feel your eyes droop heavy with sleep. Allow yourself to relax. Make yourself ready to drift into sleep. Close your eyes with the belief that you are safe and protected from your worries. Know that the only thing you need to do or get done right now is rest.

With that in mind, sleep.

7. **Drink a glass of warm turmeric milk:** The last golden rule has something to do with loving grandmothers and warm milk. Remember how your grandmother would lovingly bring you a glass of warm turmeric milk or *haldi doodh* for you before you went to sleep? Those of us who were fortunate to experience this can rest easy having known such deep love. For others, there's always turmeric milk. Drinking a glass at night before bed promotes sleep because milk has tryptophan, an amino acid which induces sleep. This allows you to sleep better.

Give these seven golden rules for sleep a go to improve your quality of sleep. These golden rules are imbued with the rich legacy of our culture and heritage. Try following them and you may find that sleep has nothing to do with white noise machines or duck feather pillows and more to do with the gentle rhythms of the mind and body or creating a sacred space for yourself where you can find sleep peacefully and easily.

Hindu scriptures assign deep sleep a status of high importance. There are various references to the right sleeping posture. A Gujarati proverb says, *'Undha sooye abhagi,seedha sooye rogi, dabba sooye sansari ane jamne sooye jogi.'* This age-old tip translates to, 'The unfortunate sleep on their stomach, the diseased and the sick on their backs. The man of the world sleeps on his left and the ascetic sleeps on his right.' What it attempts to explain is the right position for us to sleep. The proverb states that a frustrated, anxious or wearied person sleeps on their stomach, facing away from the world. The sick, the obese or those who snore loudly sleep on their backs. Sleeping on the left, or *vamakushi*, is the sleeping position recommended for householders, people who have work to do, or those who need more energy in their lives. It is believed that when you sleep on your left side, your right nostril or *suryanadi* gets activated and as a result, you get more energy to perform your daily activities.

An ascetic who is unbothered by worry sleeps on the right and their left nostril or *chandranadi* is activated. This cools the system down, quietens it and fosters detachment. For householders, although we need the energy of the *suryanadi*, we also need the calm and detachment of the *chandranadi*.

Your body knows what it needs at any point of time, so learn to listen to it and adjust your sleeping posture accordingly. Sometimes, if the temperature of the room is too low, your body will not turn to the right. It will automatically turn left. At night too, the body will automatically turn from left to right as required. It is up to you to listen. Another tip is that when you get up in the morning, turn to your right and take a few deep breaths; this let/s you cultivate *vairagya* or detachment which will help you ground or calm yourself and help you clean your bowels more easily. By doing so, you can help your body in the morning.

Are Late Nights a Problem?

Late nights have also become a cultural phenomenon and a part of our daily lives. Though Indian scriptures extol the values of sleeping early and waking up early, much of that advice is now overlooked and unheeded. We need to remember that, for over a million years, evolution has worked to align the human body with the natural cycles of day and night. We have evolved to wind down when the moon appears and rise with the glory of the emerging sun. Expecting that evolution will make our bodies adapt to our current lifestyle preferences overnight is unrealistic.

Is there anything wrong with sleeping late and waking late? Is it harmful to have late nights every day? Is there any advantage to being an early riser? Let us look consider the following points.

1. **Late nights create bad eating habits:** People who stay up late at night tend to consume more calories by eating more junk, which leads to unhealthy eating habits.
2. **Late nights weaken the immune system:** The body's hormonal levels fluctuate throughout the day, along with

other natural cycles which are affected when we try to change the body's natural clock by sleeping late. This stresses out your body which in turn leads to a weakened immune system. Remember when you had a bout of the cold or flu or felt weak and ask yourself what your sleeping habits were like during that time.

3. **What you do to your body now, your body will do to you later:** Many of us nowadays believe that we have personalized body clocks that are in tune with our bad sleeping habits. This belief in a separate body clock makes us think that it is fine to sleep late because the body is not showing any signs of weakness or harm. But nothing is further from the truth. As we discussed earlier, what we do to our bodies in our youth is what our body does to us as we grow older. Bad sleep hygiene will invariably be reflected in an array of lifestyle diseases as one ages. Remember, there is nothing like your own body clock. Everybody has a biological clock which may have a few small differences but is more or less the same. Also remember, your body is only used to your sleeping habits, or your body clock, as you call it. That is you are creating your so-called body clock through a process of repeating a bad habit.

4. **Digestion suffers:** When you sleep late, your digestive system becomes confused. Our digestive system works optimally between sunrise and sunset. When we eat late at night and keep awake till odd hours, the food is not digested completely as our system's capacities are lower at night. Many digestive enzymes are secreted in minimal quantities at night and so, when you eat heavy meals later

in the day, you are, in fact, increasing pressure on your gastrointestinal tract and the body. This is one of the main reasons why night owls and late eaters suffer from so many digestive disorders.

5. **Mental functioning weakens:** Mental functions such as creativity and awareness peak when the body is well-rested and cared for. When people work late hours, the body is denied its fair share of rest and relaxation. A direct consequence of that is a decrease in mental functioning over time.

6. **The spiritual aspect of being an early riser:** The time between 4.00 a.m. till sunrise is considered the most auspicious hour of the day. It is the time that allows us to be most closely aware of the spiritual truth of our lives as humans as it is a time of peace, quiet and clarity. Light is a symbol of knowledge. At dawn, when the sun rises, there is a lot of activity in nature; we can almost sense the awakening of life's vitality. Darkness and night, on the other hand, are considered the opposites. The night is usually associated with fatigue from the day's work and worries. Darkness also symbolizes ignorance. It is assumed that those who choose to work at night chose ignorance over knowledge and lethargy over vitality.

   Waking up early has innumerable benefits such as being proactive because you have a lot of time to plan, more time to exercise and more free time as you are not rushed. The absence of rush gives you fewer things to worry about and you are not as stressed, which improves your mental health, enhances productivity, improves your lifestyle, helps you sustain a healthier diet and so on. We must make a conscious choice of taking care of ourselves. This choice cannot be meaningfully exercised till we try to take care of our bodies. The best care we can give our bodies is by tuning into nature rather than working against her rhythms. If this is not a priority for us now, it will become a punishment for us later.

All this talk of sleep doesn't imply that one must sleep all the time. Sleep, like everything else in our life, must be balanced. Too much of a good thing turns into poison. So, how much should a person sleep? Around 3 per cent of people need less than six hours of sleep. Their bodies show no significant wear and tear or increased risk for lifestyle diseases despite the reduced sleep span. However, the other 97 per cent needs roughly eight hours of sleep every night for a healthy lifestyle. It is believed that a person experiences around five segments of sleep cycles spanning 90 minutes every night. In the first few cycles, the body concentrates on cleaning and maintaining the brain and heart. In the later cycles, the mind processes and consolidates the information it has accessed during the day, storing it for further use.

Sleep deprivation causes an increased risk of stress. It also affects memory loss and causes fatigue. Serious implications of sleep loss include diabetes, heart disease, obesity, depression and hypertension. We need to learn to listen to our body when tell-tale signs of stress or other issues begin to affect our sleep. Sleep is a basic biological need and must be given due importance. Sleep helps children focus and improve memory. Our body's innate healing capacities kick into full gear and the immune system gets revitalized during sleep. Good sleep is indispensable for your good health and to reset your life.

If all this reading has made you sleepy, I suggest you have a nap right about now so we can get to the next section happy, relaxed and well-rested.

FIVE B

The Five Circles of Food

Anna he purna Brahma.

Food defines a lot of who we are as people. For instance, we would know a little something about a person who enjoys his undhiyu or her gaathiyas or their parathas or a person who raves about his dosa and filter coffee. In any country, food is an essential part of culture and identity. In India, it shows who is a Gujarati, Bengali, Tamilian or Punjabi. Think about it your earliest memories of getting ready for school and hurriedly gulping down the hot breakfast your mother made with a lot of love. Think of how any festival we celebrate is coloured by the food we eat. Could you imagine Ganesh Chaturthi without ladoos and modaks or Diwali without the plethora of sweets that we enjoy? As a country, we are truly blessed with a rich heritage of food that dates back centuries ago. Our culinary traditions stem from the scriptures imbued with rich variations across regions. Each part of the country contributes to our culinary legacy, bringing with it a cornucopia of fresh local produce, spices, condiments, utensils, techniques and styles.

Philosophically too, it is also one of the four pillars of yoga: *ahar*, *vihar*, *achar* and *vichar*. For instance, 'ahar' in

Sanskrit doesn't simply connote what we eat; it also connotes sustenance. Ahar, in its truest sense, is that which sustains us or nourishes us, how much of it we eat, how we eat, the attitude we have or the mood we are in when we are eating. All this is very important and makes a vast difference in our lives.

After all, we are what we eat. Yet, the lives we lead now have somehow separated us from food as a source of joy and nourishment for us. It has become a constant source of worry. Folks obsessed with weight loss nowadays count calories because they are obsessed with weight loss. Weight loss is not the same thing as a healthy body. And food should never be seen as something that harms you or worries you, especially in a country with such a rich, culinary legacy. There is something to be said about the joy of eating in our lives. With that, let's look at the **five circles of food.** As you enter each circle, you will know a little more about the food you eat and by the end of it, you have reset your relationship with food and also begun to savour the joy of eating and the joy of food.

But before we enter the circles of food, let us learn a little more about the place where all the food we eat goes—our stomach.

Did you know that our stomach is also called our second brain? Scientists call it the enteric nervous system or ENS. It consists of two thin layers of more than 100 million nerve cells lining our gastrointestinal tract from the oesophagus to the rectum. Though the ENS can't form thoughts as our brain can, there is much back-and-forth communication between the brain and the gut, enough that scientists speak of a definite connection. The ENS's main role is controlling digestion, from swallowing and the release of enzymes that break down food to the control of blood flow which helps with nutrient absorption and elimination.

We certainly have many expressions in our language that attest to the same, such as 'I simply could not stomach it,' for when we cannot accept a situation, or 'I have butterflies in my stomach' for when we are excited or nervous. And who has not experienced a sudden urge to go to the bathroom right before an important event like an exam or a presentation? Our mind and our gut are very connected and if we listened to our gut for that 'gut feeling' more often, we would be better off.

Why is good gut health important? Well, firstly, it helps us feel better, lighter and undisturbed during the day. Good gut health also means good mental health. How does this work? While scientists thought for decades that the brain mainly controls the gut, it is the other way round: Instead of anxiety and depression, for example, contributing to digestive ailments like irritable bowel syndrome (IBS), constipation, diarrhoea, bloating, pain and an upset stomach, it is actually poor gut health that might cause anxiety and depression or poor mental health in general. Poor gut health increases inflammation and causes hyperarousal of the stress pathways, causing anxiety and a 'fight or flight' reaction or the release of neurotoxins that can cause brain fog and fatigue. It is vital to keep our gut happy and healthy through a balanced diet.

But what is gut health exactly? There are certainly signs when one's gut is healthy: regular and adequate bowel movements at least once a day (preferably right in the morning after getting up) is one such sign. Also, the absence of abdominal symptoms like gas, bloating or abdominal pain.

Now we are ready for the food circles. Let's go all in.

The First Food Circle—Know Your Food

Food, at its heart, is energy. Traditionally, it is believed that there are three types of energies: *tamasic* or dull energy, *rajasic* or active energy and *satvik* or balanced energy. These three energies are always present in all of us, but in different proportions. Each form of energy has its own purpose. For example, a bit of dull energy is required for adequate rest and sleep, while active energy is necessary for work and balanced energy is needed for fulfilling aspirations in life. Makes sense, doesn't it? Food, it is believed, directly impacts the proportions of these energies in our body because the food we eat impacts us on a physical, emotional, mental and spiritual level. Let's understand what each type of food is and how it impacts our body, mind and mood.

An action-inducing diet mainly consists of *rajasic* food i.e., it contains spices and anything rich in taste such as onion, garlic, fried food, coffee, tea, refined food and chocolates. This food gives us instant energy for a brief period. Thus, a diet dominated by pungent or oily food or energizing substances, such as tea and coffee, fall into this category. When consumed in moderation or when you are going to have a strenuous day full of physical activity, this kind of food serves as an instant source of energy. But in the long run, they are often addictive and disturb the mind-body equilibrium. This type of diet feeds the body at the cost of the mind. Over a period of time, a person on this kind of diet exhibits a weak digestive system, is always in a rush to eat and prefers rich foods.

At the other end of the spectrum is a diet full of dull energy or a *tamasic* diet. Such a diet mainly consists of reheated or chemically processed food such as eggs, cheese and meat—anything packaged, really—and alcohol and cigarettes. These foods may be easy to eat and prepare but they do not give us much energy; on the contrary, they take a long time to digest, using up precious energy that could have been spent on some other bodily or mental functions. Accordingly, a person on such a diet will be dull, unimaginative, unmotivated, careless, unaware and lethargic. Often, they may experience illnesses such as diabetes, obesity and liver disease.

That leaves satvik or pure food. Food that is easy to digest and does not require much energy from the body to process. A satvik diet is not bland or tasteless. As you will see at the end of the chapter, it is full of taste and variety. All you need is to be willing to put in a little bit of effort to make some small changes in your habits for your well-being! A balanced diet is a diet that includes seasonal fresh fruits and vegetables, whole grains, pulses, sprouts, dried nuts, seeds, honey, fresh herbs, milk and dairy products. The satvik process starts long before eating as satvik food is prepared, cooked and eaten with love, gratitude and awareness.

This kind of food raises the satva element in us or in our consciousness levels. It also makes our nervous system work better. A satvik person is calm, peaceful, serene, amicable and full of energy, enthusiasm, health, hope, aspirations and creativity—an overall balanced personality. Another advantage of a satvik diet is that it helps to keep one's weight in check, in addition to working wonders for your skin and hair.

Now let's enter the **second food circle**.

The Second Food Circle—Building Blocks

Food is the source of the building blocks of our body. Let's take a closer look at each one of them.

Proteins

Proteins are large complex molecules composed of amino acids and are necessary for the chemical processes of the body. As structural compounds, they are the body's building blocks and necessary for growth and for repairing and building tissue. There are two types of proteins: simple ones composed only of amino acids and conjugated proteins that, in addition to an amino group, are also contained in prosthetic groups, i.e. a group of carbohydrates, lipids, pigments, etc.

How much protein should we consume in a day? A rough guide is that a fourth of each plate should be made up of proteins. That means we should consume proteins with every single meal! The recommended dietary allowance to prevent deficiency for an average sedentary adult is roughly a gram per kilogram of body weight—for a sixty-kilogram person, that would be sixty grams of protein a day, or for an eighty-kilogram person, about eight grams and so on.

What foods are good sources of protein? Beans, peas, lentils, sabja (chia seeds), dairy products, nuts and nut butters (such as peanut butter), soybean and tofu are good vegetarian sources of protein.

Fats

Fats have long gotten a bad reputation and low-fat diets have been propagated for decades. However, the body needs essential fats—you may have heard of omega-3 and omega-6 fatty acids. They are found in foods like almonds, avocados, coconut milk, flaxseeds and flaxseed oil, *sabja*, walnuts and walnut oil, canola oil, soybean oil, mustard oil, sunflower oil and tofu.

A big advantage of having adequate fats with every meal (about a couple of tablespoons) is that fats do not affect our blood sugar levels. While carbs will do that and you will experience a 'sugar high' after eating carbs (and then a low), fats keep the blood sugar level balanced. This is important for diabetics, for example, who can experience an improvement in their condition by following a high-fat, low-carb diet.

Carbohydrates

Food contains three types of carbohydrates: sugar, starches and fibres. Carbohydrates are either simple or complex, depending on the food's chemical structure and how quickly sugar is digested and absorbed. Carbohydrate-rich food is usually what we call junk food—processed cereal, canned juices, soda, fried foods . . . you get the idea. Note that, unlike the essential fats and proteins that the body needs, there are no essential carbohydrates. If we eat a balanced diet as suggested above, we will get enough carbohydrates that we need for energy without making an effort.

Micronutrients

As seen above, nutrients like proteins, fats, carbohydrates, vitamins and minerals are the substances in food that drive biological activity. They are essential for the human body and perform vital functions. Two of them—vitamins and minerals—are called micronutrients. Though the body needs them only in small amounts (microdoses) their impact on the body's health is critical and a deficiency in any of them can cause severe, even life-threatening conditions. Often, deficiencies may be less critical and thus, less notable but they will hinder us from living life to the fullest of our capacity. For example, we might experience a reduction in energy levels, mental clarity and overall capacity. A healthy and balanced diet can prevent most of these deficiencies.

Vitamins

There are 13 essential vitamins for the human body (*vita* in Latin means 'life')—vitamins A, C, D, E, K and the eight B vitamins i.e., thiamine, riboflavin, niacin, pantothenic acid, biotin, B6, B12 and folate. Vitamins are nutritionally essential organic substances that play a catalytic role in cell metabolism. They promote overall health by preventing degenerative diseases. Particularly essential vitamins are vitamins A, B-complex, C, D, E and K. We need to make sure to provide our body with a daily dose of all vitamins through our food.

Vitamin A is largely found in vegetables and fruits. Carrots are also a chief source of vitamin A. It is necessary for proper and correct vision and a deficiency can result in night blindness, weakness in the eyes, defective bone and teeth formation and poor general growth. The average intake should not exceed 4000-5000 International Units (IU). Excess of vitamin A produces toxic conditions in the body, blurred vision and headaches in adults, nervous irritability in infants, nausea, coarsening and loss of hair, drying and scaling of the skin, bone pain, fatigue and drowsiness.

The important vitamins within the **B-complex** are B1, B2, B6 and B12. **B1**, also called thiamine, is most abundant in cereal grains and certain seeds. The recommended daily intake is 1.2 milligrams (mg) for men and 1.1 mg for women. For pregnant or lactating women, the amount is 1.4 mg daily. Deficiency of B1 may cause beriberi, a disease characterized by multiple neuritis, general debility and painful rigidity.

B2, also called riboflavin, functions as part of the metabolic system. It is most abundant in whey and the recommended average daily intake is 1.2-1.7 mg. A deficiency of B2 is characterized by symptoms including a reddening of the lips, ocular disturbances and inflammations of the skin.

B6 functions in the formation and break down of protein in living tissues. It is particularly abundant in yeast and certain cereal grains and the recommended average daily intake is 2-2.2 mg. Deficiency results in issues such as skin erosions, which the vitamin usually prevents.

B12 accelerates the digestive process and helps in the assimilation of nutrients. It is found in milk and not more than 3-4 micrograms per day are needed to prevent symptoms of deficiencies such as defective functioning of the intestine, constipation or diarrhoea. Note that there are no plant-based sources of B12 and those who follow a vegan diet need to supplement this essential vitamin!

Vitamin C is important for a host of functions. It is essential to many metabolic functions such as the synthesis of a protein called collagen, the maintenance of the structural strength of blood vessels, the metabolism of certain amino acids and the synthesis or release of hormones in the adrenal glands. It also helps in the prevention of the common cold and bacterial infections. Vitamin C is largely found in lime, citrus fruits, fresh vegetables and fruits like guavas and strawberries. The recommended average daily intake is 90 mg a day for men and 75 mg a day for women or 120 mg during pregnancy.

Vitamin D helps in the intestinal absorption of calcium and other metabolic processes. It is found in milk and sunlight and may not need to be ingested in regions which offer sufficient sunlight coverage. However, in some regions, a reverse trend of vitamin D deficiency is often observed due to a general avoidance of the sun! The recommended daily vitamin D intake is for adults older than nineteen years old is 600 IU. Deficiency causes rickets, a condition that causes bone deficiency in children and 'soft bones' in adults. Since this vitamin is stored in the body if taken in excess, it produces toxic conditions including weakness, fatigue, loss of appetite, nausea, vomiting and growth failure in children.

Vitamin E is said to have an active role in prolonging one's life span and reducing the risk of coronary diseases. It is useful in the treatment of numerous diseases, especially muscular dystrophy and is an excellent antioxidant. It is found mainly in cereals or vegetable oils and occurs abundantly in wheat germ. The recommended daily intake is 15 mg but varies depending on age and constitution. A deficiency of this vitamin can produce chronic defects concerning fat absorption in premature infants and older persons.

Vitamin K is important for the healthy coagulation of blood. It is found in green plants and leafy vegetables. The recommended daily intake is 120 micrograms (mcg) for men and 90 mcg for women. A deficiency will manifest as an increase in the time taken for blood to clot. Vitamin K is also used as a food preservative to prevent fermentation.

Minerals

Minerals are important for several body processes. Iron is needed to make haemoglobin; deficiencies in iron result in anaemia. Sodium and potassium are important for maintaining homeostasis, i.e., the overall functioning of the bodily systems. Excess sodium increases blood pressure while too little may cause epileptic seizures and low blood pressure. Loss of potassium through diarrhoea may result in loss of tissue excitability and muscle paralysis. Iodine is needed to synthesize thyroid hormones. Minerals are found in abundance in green leafy vegetables, fresh fruits, milk and milk products.

Yogic and ayurvedic schools of thought suggest diseases originate from wrong eating habits and recommend a balanced diet. A balanced diet, in other words, of cereals, legumes, vegetables, salads, milk products, dry fruits and honey—the five traditional food groups which can go a long way in ensuring a long, healthy life.

There are five traditional, basic food groups that provide a balanced diet—cereals, legumes, salads, vegetables, fruits and nuts, milk products and jaggery or honey. These assure a steady supply of all building blocks and should be included in one's daily diet. We will quickly go over some information highlights of the five food groups.

In wholegrains of rice and wheat, the vital outer covering of these grains is conserved. This covering is necessary for growth. Among vegetables, green herbs such as *bhindi* (okra), *baingan* (aubergine), *parwal* (snake gourd), *karela* (bitter gourd) and *palak* (spinach) have high mineral and vitamin content and nutritional value. Among legumes, *moong dal* (green lentils) is easily digestible, even if a person is of advanced age. Sprouted *moong* enhances its nutritional value and increases its volume. *Chana* (Bengal gram or chickpeas) and other heavier pulses and beans are more suitable for those who engage in heavy physical labour than those with sedentary lifestyles.

Salads are a must with every meal as they provide the requisite minerals and vitamins for daily dietary requirements. Among salads, lettuce leaves, carrots, beetroot and others are beneficial. If such vegetables are not easily available, leafy vegetables do the trick and herbs like mint, parsley or basil count as green leafy vegetables. They are wonderful sources of vitamins, minerals and fibre, so make sure to include them in your diet plans.

Fruits are also a must in the daily diet. They provide fructose after being converted into glucose—a preferred source of energy for the body—and are easily digestible. Note that all fruits that you consume should be properly ripened.

Until the age of twenty-five, milk helps the body grow. After this age, we need milk products less. Curd, however, is a stomach pacifier that neutralizes acidity and helps in digestion and elimination. Compared to milk, it offers double the benefits as the bacteria in yoghurt—*lactobacillus, bulgaricus* and *streptocus thermophilus*—are not normally found in the digestive tract. They detoxify hostile bacteria and support existing *lactobacillus acidophilus* and *bifidobacterium*.

Research has proven that regular consumption of curd prevents stomach ulcers and cures diarrhoea and constipation. However, be aware that storebought curd does not usually contain the curative bifidobacterium (also known as *bifidus*) or *lactobacillus acidophilus*, which is why it is better to make curd at home.

Dry fruits are excellent protein and vitamin supplements but must be consumed in small quantities. Almonds, cashews, walnuts, peanuts and other nuts may be included in breakfast or evening snacks.

Refined sugar devitalizes the body as it passes through many chemical processes and is considered to have anti-calcium properties. Thus, use brown sugar instead, or jaggery, a dark brown sugar made from the sap of the palm tree; it is an excellent source of iron. You could also use honey.

What Does the Ideal Plate Look Like?

In terms of the ideal plate of food as we prepare it, half of it should consist of vegetables, preferably non-starchy ones. One-fourth should consist of a protein source, such as pulses and legumes. Healthy carbohydrates—as found in starchy vegetables or grains—should consist of another one-fourth of the plate. The plate should be rounded off by a healthy serving of fats such as a couple of tablespoons of oil or ghee. Alternatively, you could opt for a handful of nuts and seeds or even fruits like coconut and avocado. Remember to stick to these proportions for all meals to make sure you do justice to each of the essential food groups.

The Third Food Circle—Knowing How Much to Eat

We should spend some time thinking about how much food we actually need. Should we eat until our stomach bursts? No. Should we be perpetually hungry or unsatisfied? Certainly not. The five circles of food will help you understand that food is not your enemy and they will help you reset your relationship with food. You must understand that is not food that makes you gain weight, but your habits around food to begin resetting your relationship with it.

How much is the right amount when it comes to food? Yogic and ayurvedic schools of thought believe that less is more when it comes to a healthy diet. This does not mean that you have to starve or never eat the things you love ever again. It means you must know your body and help it as opposed to overloading it with too much food. A good rule of thumb is that when you eat, eat only till you are half-full. The next one quarter should be filled with water, and the last quarter should be empty. That is right! A quarter of our stomach should be empty at all times, not filled with desserts or any such sweet temptations when we are already full. Do not be fearful that you will go hungry. The point of this exercise is to ensure that the food you have already consumed will get digested and you should feel hungry again, at which point you should have a small portion of a healthy snack or fruit. Following this rule will give you more variety to enjoy rather than stifling your cravings with strict, unpractical diets that have no connection to your life or food heritage.

And how do we know when we are full? Should we start counting calories and follow complicated charts based on our height, weight, age and activity? Certainly not. Though diet and cooking can be a science, we should not get lost in it or get too preoccupied. Do not make your health or diet a fetish, but do not neglect it either. As a general rule of thumb, eat when you are hungry, drink when you are thirsty and stop eating a little before you feel satiated. As you can see, it is more important to listen to our own body and find out what it needs than to count calories.

Simple!

In this context, the question that often comes up is if fasting is a good habit or not. Though yoga does not advocate fasting per se as it weakens the body, much can certainly be said about detoxing. Detoxing the body at regular intervals is a must and we can easily do that by including a day in the month when we only eat fruits. We should ideally opt for whole and fresh seasonal fruits (not just juice) to take full advantage of natural dietary fibre which is good for our digestion and to clear our system, making us feel light, fresh and renewed.

Let's take a quick look at the notion of skipping a meal, shall we?

I often hear comments such as, 'I had no time for breakfast,' 'I forgot to eat,' or 'I don't feel like cooking for just one person.' This is a cruel thing to do to your body.

Let's consider what happens physically when you skip a meal. Many people believe that skipping a meal will help them lose weight as they are giving the body fewer calories, but this is not true. In fact, quite the opposite happens. When we skip or have long gaps between meals, the body goes into starvation mode since it doesn't know when the next meal will come. As a result, once that next meal comes, the calories not needed for immediate processing are stored as fat reserves for the next round of 'starvation'.

So, you see that by skipping meals or being irregular with food or food timings, the body enters a mode of self-preservation under the belief that something abnormal is occurring. Naturally, this also affects our minds—a lack of food can make us feel irritable, short-tempered or argumentative and we may even get headaches. In addition, we lack concentration since we are distracted by hunger and unable to focus on the tasks at hand.

The Fourth Circle of Food—How Should We Eat?

Now, this may sound like a silly question: How should we eat?

'We put the food in our mouth, chew and swallow!' you may respond. But it is not that easy since there are many habits we have picked up along the way that sabotage the process of eating food.

For instance, many of us have a habit of gulping down our food or eating on the run while walking or standing. This is wrong. Whenever you eat or drink something, sit down and take the time to eat and chew properly. Otherwise, eating while walking or talking means we swallow a lot of air with our food, which causes gas and indigestion. The body and the mind need to be stable when consuming anything.

Another habit we have, especially if we like the food, is eating quickly and greedily. We eat in big bites, taking the next bite before the previous one has been fully chewed. That is another wrong and unhealthy habit because digestion starts in the mouth—Eat slowly and chew each mouthful of food thoroughly at least ten times. Finish each bite before preparing the next one to put in your mouth.

Milk and juices are liquid foods and should not be gulped down like water. By following the saying, 'chew the liquids and drink the solids,' you will relieve your stomach of a lot of work because the digestive process starts right inside your mouth. You may feel tempted to wash down every bite with a sip of water, but yogic and ayurvedic philosophy advises against doing so since it dilutes the gastric juices required for digestion. Drink water about half an hour before your meal and wait until about half an hour after the meal to drink again.

Food tastes better in the company of friends, no doubt, but that does not mean we have to talk incessantly while eating; we could also just eat food in silence while enjoying the presence of others. After all, anything important can be discussed after the meal. Do not talk too much while eating and take care to avoid becoming agitated over anything since doing so would use up much of the energy needed for the stomach's work.

Last but not least, do not eat more than you absolutely need to. Try to finish your meal when you feel you could still eat a little more.

The Fifth Circle of Food—What Should We Not Eat?

This may seem counterintuitive in a chapter on food. But it isn't. The knowledge of anything is incomplete if you do not also understand the other side of things. If you need to know how to eat right, it is vital to know what not to eat. Even if you forget every other circle, keep this section in mind so it can be the start of your healthy food journey.

Research shows that fragmentation of whole foods destroys nutrients and lessens their suitability as a part of the diet. Whole carrots contain more nutrients than carrot juice, brown rice is more nutritional than polished rice and whole wheat is more nutritional than wheat germ, for example. Thus, the overall nutritional effect of whole foods as compared to processed, fragmented, or refined foods is far superior.

At first glance, fragmented foods may seem more nourishing than whole foods. Dried apricots, for example, have a higher percentage of calcium and iron than fresh apricots. But this is due to the extraction of water which triples or quadruples the number of fruits per pound, thereby increasing more nutrients per pound. For a true comparison, however, we must compare each fruit, namely one dried apricot to one fresh one. Using this method, we will find that fresh apricots contain both a higher percentage (and a wider range) of nutrients.

Another example is whey, the liquid that remains after milk has been curdled and strained. However, as a by-product, powdered whey is but a nutritional shadow of whole milk. Processing in general causes a drastic amount of nutrient loss as a result of heat, oxidation, chemicals and enzymatic destruction. It is correct to say that the foods have been 'devitalized'. Only whole, natural foods contain the appropriately proportionate amount of nutrients that the body requires, making whole natural foods the ideal food group to help develop optimum health. The fact remains that extracts or concentrates are universally inferior compared to the whole natural foods they represent.

Raw Food

Raw food, such as seasonal fruits and fresh vegetables, add fibre to your meals. Fibre helps you feel satiated faster, reducing the amount you eat and helping you with your bowel movement. They also allow your body to access vitamins and minerals in fruits and vegetables unaffected by heat or oxidation. Cooking adversely affects water-soluble vitamins (such as ascorbic and pantothenic acids), lowering the vitamin content of food and modifying vitamin rations, which are important elements of organic foods. Cooking may render soluble minerals less usable and some may escape into the air as gases (particularly sulphur and iodine). Cooking softens vegetable fibre, which may hamper intestinal motility and promote fermentation and putrefaction. In terms of proteins, cooking removes an amino group from an amino acid or another compound, making them more difficult to digest. Heat also changes fats to toxic hydrocarbons and free fatty acids, both of which are highly irritating. Heated fats and oils have also been shown in countless experiments to be highly carcinogenic.

It is thus advisable to increase your intake of raw salads and fruits and to be gentle when cooking your food. Say no to high-temperature cooking or microwave cooking.

Plant-Based Diet

Studies have shown that a plant-based diet lowers the risk of diabetes, high blood pressure, ischemic heart disease (problems caused by narrowed heart arteries) and strokes.

Red meat and processed meat have been shown to metabolize into toxins that cause damage to our blood vessels and other organs, which can potentially exacerbate the risk of heart disease and diabetic conditions.

A plant-based diet also appears to lead to lower low-density lipoprotein cholesterol levels, lower blood pressure, lower rates of hypertension, lower body mass index, lower overall risk of cancer and a generally lower risk of chronic disease. This doesn't mean you have to give up on food that you love. Just try to be more inclusive and accepting of plant-based diets or try to include at least one plant-based item in all meals.

Always take it one step at a time.

Caffeine

As a stimulant of the central nervous system, too much caffeine damages the body by overstimulating the nervous system over an extended period of consumption. In time, these symptoms give way to chronic fatigue, lack of energy and persistent insomnia. Caffeinated beverages can irritate the stomach lining and can cause the stomach to excrete excess acids, producing a rebound effect. This aggravates ulcers and other stomach problems. Caffeine also has a constricting effect on blood vessels and can interfere with digestion and high doses of caffeine can even induce vomiting. Caffeine has also been found to interfere with calcium and iron absorption, resulting in anaemia.

Does caffeine give one a surge of energy? Yes, because it raises blood sugar levels, which along with mind-stimulating action, produces increased energy. While this seems desirable, increased blood sugar levels draws out the insulin response, which not only cancels this surge but produces a drop in energy levels.

The bottom line is: don't overdo your chai and coffee intake. Try to stick to a maximum of two cups a day; don't pump a constant flood of caffeine into your body just because you're overworked or need to study for any exam.

Alcohol

Alcohol falls under the category of *tamasic* food as it makes the body and mind dull and lethargic. It also acts as a drug and when consumed in excess, can damage the liver or lead to addiction. If you want to be addicted, be addicted to your life, your goals and your aspirations. That is more intoxicating and does not give you a hangover the next day!

Tobacco

Though not a food per se, tobacco products like cigarettes and other nicotine products are popularly 'enjoyed' worldwide. While it temporarily stimulates the lungs and circulation, it is *tamasic* in nature as it fosters addiction, weakens the lungs and poses the risk of cancer.

In short, food should ideally be easy to eat and easy to digest in its natural, unheated and unprocessed state. It should offer a broad variety of nutrients, a moderate amount of fibre, leave behind an alkaline ash after metabolism that aids in the removal of impurities and be free of irritants and substances that make digestion more difficult.

And there you have it—the five circles to reset your relationship with food. Now, before we turn to some appetizing diet plans to guide you further, let us take a quick look at the question of overeating.

Overeating vs Moderation and Discipline

The size of our stomach is roughly the size of our hand. That is not much, right? How much food can fit into this area? When one overeats, the size of the stomach gets distended or inflated and thus, will demand food in excess. Ideally, one should eat only till the stomach is half-full, leaving a quarter for gases to form and a quarter for liquids. Liquids should be had half an hour before or after a meal so as not to dilute the gastric juices that help in digestion.

There is a story of King Prasenajit, the king of the land of Kosala which was located north-east of the Indian subcontinent during Buddha's time. He used to eat a bucketful of rice and curry and afterwards, fall asleep and snore during Buddha's discourses. Buddha advised him to eat one lesser mouthful of food each day and the following day, two lesser mouthfuls of food and so on. Prasenajit followed this advice and over time, became slim and could even ride his horse again.

Overeating makes all the organs work very hard, aggravating many diseases like heart disease, diabetes and orthopaedic problems, even causing premature death. Therefore, one should wisely reduce one's food intake if one is overeating.

How much food should we eat? There is a saying: eat like a king in the morning, like a prince in the afternoon and like a pauper in the evening. This adage still holds true; we should be starting our day with a good, healthy breakfast and ideally, this meal should be the heaviest of the day because we have the whole day to work it off. Also, we need energy for all the different activities we must do over the course of the next sixteen hours or so—get up, carry out our morning routines, go to work or school, do our daily chores, follow a hobby and most importantly, keep our spirits up. This requires energy and as we have seen earlier, a large part of this energy comes from our food.

Did you know that a good breakfast is one of the best immunity boosters? A good breakfast can instigate our immune system to optimize our natural defences against infection, including fighting viruses that cause respiratory illnesses like the common cold, flu and even COVID-19.

Lunch should be taken in moderate quantities. It should sustain us, but we should not feel full and sluggish afterwards—that is a sign that we have eaten too much. The right kind of food should never make you feel tired, gaseous or bloated; you should feel energized and alert after a balanced meal. If you feel listless after your meal, you need to examine the quantity and quality of your food and make some changes.

Then, we have dinner—for most, it is the biggest and most important meal of the day and one that often has a social component. Dinner is when the family gets together and everyone is done rushing around. However, it is also often when it is almost time to sleep. Think about this—your system is calming down, preparing for the night and you give it the heaviest meal of the day just because it is convenient for you to eat at that time. But what about your system that has been serving you so faithfully the whole day?

During the day, food has to be converted into energy and this energy is used for activity. At night, one has no need this energy and so, at bedtime, one should not sleep after consuming a heavy meal since unnecessary toxins and gases might be created. So after this heavy meal at the end of the day, you feel tired and maybe you engage in a sedentary activity before retiring to bed. There could also be complaints of acidity, hiccups or a sense of heaviness, followed by fitful sleep or difficulty in falling asleep in the first place. This is because your system is busy digesting the large amount of food you fed it just a while ago.

This is detrimental across three levels: firstly, the various systems of the body cannot fulfil their duties, which are regeneration and rest at night; secondly, the sleep gets disturbed because of the activity going on internally, making deep rest impossible; thirdly, the system becomes sluggish and digests food slowly, often until the next morning, potentially causing it to signal that it is still full and not yet ready for the next meal. As a result, we might skip breakfast, which is the most important part of the day and a vicious cycle starts—characterized by insufficient or slow digestion and irregularity in food habits. Eating meals in a rushed frame of mind and cravings for snacks or quick fixes rather than proper meals also starts this vicious cycle. It is best to always eat with a relaxed frame of mind and if possible, the last meal should be had around dusk.

Some Tips for Mindful and Conscious Eating

Yoga advocates for moderation and discipline in meals. It is important to maintain a mindful attitude while cooking or eating so that the right energy flows into the meal that we prepare. But are we even conscious and aware when we eat our food? In fact, very often, we seem to be hurrying and rushing through our meals. We are unmindful of what we eat, how we eat, or how much we eat. The simplest test is to ask a person what they had for dinner the previous day. Very often, they may have forgotten what they ate.

Food should be eaten slowly and in a good frame of mind. Always prefer fresh food since food cooked and stored in the fridge loses its vitality and degenerates, making us dull and lethargic.

Canned and preserved food has lower nutritional value and the added danger of chemicals. Thus, one should avoid canned and preserved food as far as possible.

The same is true for fried food since excess oil increases the cholesterol levels of arteries and over time, the accumulation of excess cholesterol causes the arteries to become narrower and narrower, eventually hampering the flow of blood. Those suffering from coronary disease should avoid fried food completely as it can block the coronary arteries. Instead, steamed food and vegetables are a better option.

It is also very necessary to be mindful of the climatic conditions to determine what we should eat and what not. For example, in the monsoon, it is not desirable or advisable to eat too much of a liquid diet or partake in heavy meals. The mistake of eating ice cream in winter is also obvious— our system already has to work hard than in summer to keep our body temperature up; why make it harder by eating something cold that your body will have to heat up rather than something warm or at room temperature? In addition, ice cream can cool our throats and cause a cold or sore throat.

Likewise, food that contributes to generating heat in our body should be avoided during the summer, such as too much mango or papaya. But we do not think along these lines. Greater mindfulness is needed when it comes to considering our dietary habits.

Another aspect to consider is how we may experience various emotions while eating—anger, anxiety, or sadness. We may also be busy talking while eating and in the process, neglect to do full justice to the food being consumed. What is recommended is eating with a calm and cheerful mind. Once finished, give your system a few minutes to start the digestion process by sitting upright, eyes closed and resting for a while, or by taking a short walk after the meal instead of hurrying back to work.

Overconsumption: Comfort Eating and Social Obligations

Often, we are not hungry but if food appears before us (in a restaurant, in someone's home, at work), we tend to eat, regardless of if we are actually hungry or not. Often, we want to be polite and not refuse food that is placed in front of us, even if we are full. We can see that there is more to food than its physical properties; there is a whole emotional connection.

If someone comes to our home, as good hosts, we offer food; in casual conversation, we ask if the other person has had breakfast, lunch, or dinner yet; if someone is upset, we may offer food as consolation. Similarly, for any happy occasion—be it a wedding, an anniversary, passing exams, getting a new job, buying a new car or a new home—we distribute sweets. We learn as children that food is to be shared, that food can be had when we are happy but also when we are sad. Eating when you are emotionally stressed is referred to as 'comfort eating'—using food to comfort us when we are upset or unbalanced. It implies the usage of food to gain control over at least one aspect of our life; a life that seems terribly random and out of our control. Eating disorders are often based on this aspect—taking control of something in an otherwise unmanageable world.

However, doing so means giving in to our emotions and relying on food to address our difficult emotions. This should not be so because food can become an aspect of our life that helps in our self-improvement. Every day, three or four times, the mind can be calibrated through the consumption of food. Mealtimes become an opportunity for growth and self-discipline, when we determine how much we eat, what we eat, how we eat and with what attitude. This can help us foster a sense of control in our life in a far more positive way. Cultivating a feeling of gratitude before eating, meals at fixed times every day, not talking too much while consuming and eating in good company are some of the techniques that can be used to control the mind, keeping us alert and aware.

We should bear in mind, however, that control over food is not the end. The goal of yoga is not control over food, but rather, control over the mind. As one achieves more and more control over the mind, one automatically achieves control over food, sleep, speech and other activities. Cultivating the right attitude is important, so why not make the effort to do so?

At the other end of the spectrum of extremes, there is the fad of diets. If we know what to eat and what is the right kind of food that will make us feel healthy and balanced, why don't we eat it?

Further, we have already established that there is an emotional component to eating and there are many obstacles that the human mind must overcome before doing something, for instance, laziness. Healthy food takes time and effort; processed food does not. We simply open the fridge or open a bag of something and we feel satiated for a while.

Another obstacle is stubbornness. Sometimes when we are told to do something and we don't feel like doing it or just to be contrary, we do the exact opposite. That is why dieting does not work—the moment we are told we can only eat A, B and C and not X, Y and Z, we desire X, Y and Z more strongly than ever! Our mind latches on to what we are not supposed to have and becomes obsessed with it and then, the cravings become too intense to combat.

What must one do in such cases? We could relax the rules of not eating certain foods and tell our minds that while A, B and C are the good foods to eat, it is okay to eat X, Y and Z too—in moderation. By doing so, much of the pressure is taken off our minds and X, Y and Z move from the 'forbidden' foods area to the 'once in a while' area and out of the cravings zone. Isn't that smart?

A word about cravings: Observe yourself carefully and track when you have cravings. Quite often, rather than being triggered by certain events (a stressful exam or presentation, a new job, etc.) cravings are tied to eating too little of one or more of the essential building blocks. Protein and essential fats especially are often neglected and can cause us to reach for foods with carbohydrates instead, which causes blood sugar levels to fluctuate. If it is low, we crave sweets. But did you know that the essential fats found in nuts, seeds, fatty fruits and vegetables do not affect our blood sugar levels? The next time you have a craving for sweets, have some nuts or nut butters instead and observe what happens. You will notice that over time, your cravings will lessen, especially if you make sure to also eat adequate proteins with every single meal.

In a Nutshell: The Dos and Don'ts of a Balanced Diet

Dos

- Start your day with a good breakfast.
- Eat every four hours.
- Eat a balanced diet that includes all the food groups in the right proportions.
- Drink lime juice or have a piece of fruit if hungry between meals.
- Eat when you are in a good mood.
- Have a glass of warm water after a meal to aid digestion and flush out toxins.
- Eat more fruits and vegetables.
- Make changes to your diet gradually.

Don'ts

- Never eat in a hurry.
- Don't skip meals.
- Never eat out of frustration or when upset.
- Avoid fried food.
- Avoid going on fad diets or crash diets.
- Avoid fasting, i.e., going long intervals without food.
- Don't have your heaviest meal in the evening.
- Don't go to sleep on a full stomach.

Asanas for Better Living

'Asanas bring perfection in body, beauty in form, grace, strength, compactness and the harness and brilliance of diamonds.'

—Anonymous

Asana Practice

After sleep and food, physical movement or *asana practice* is the third important foundation of well-being. If you are sceptical about this, ask yourself what would you be able to do if you did not have the support of a healthy body. Try to remember all the times a bout of the common cold or a headache has brought you to your knees. You must understand this: despite all the smart gadgets we use, we are only as functional as the state of our bodies. Our bodies, for one thing, were not designed to sit for prolonged hours. The human body was made to move, have an erect spine and strengthen its muscles, amongst other things. But the increasingly sedentary nature of our lifestyles has meant that we are usually facing one screen or the other. As we spend hours bent over our gadgets, our spines curve, our muscles become loosened, our arteries get choked and we accumulate heaps and heaps of visceral fat on all our organs. The shift in the nature of our work implies that there is no escaping a sedentary lifestyle. For a moment, think of how vastly different the kind of work you do is from the kind of work your grandparents did. Make a simple mental list of how many times your grandparents would move during the day and how many times you move during the day. You will see how drastic the change in lifestyles has been and how much more of a sedentary lifestyle you lead.

Within no time, things have changed rapidly. For instance, did you have a smartphone when you were growing up? You can see how much our gadgets have restricted our movements. However, the awareness of this change has not really caught up with us. Before the era of gadgets, our daily life factored in a far greater range of movements, which exercised various muscles of the body and fulfilled the daily quota of movements. This helped the body achieve many vital functions such as hormone regulation, homeostasis, improved cardiovascular health, muscle growth, strengthening and so on and so forth. In your grandparent's time, many aspects of health and exercise were naturally balanced by the kind of active lives they led. This ensured that the body's natural capabilities functioned at optimal levels, which is not the case now with our increasingly sedentary lifestyles. Since times have changed, we must make a conscious effort for the sake of our bodily health. The situation demands that we make a concerted and consistent effort to take time out to physically move the body.

Just because our bodies continue to function, we assume that everything is okay. That is not so. A lack of movement and physical activity in your daily life affects you physically, physiologically and even emotionally. Repeated studies have shown that exercise releases endorphins; the body's happy hormones. These reduce your stress and anxiety levels and the amount of cortisol, a stress hormone, in your body. When you exercise, you release these happy hormones which relaxes your body and improves the functioning of your organs and systems. Why wouldn't you do something that is so good for you? If you need a little help with beginning an exercise routine, then this book is the right place to start.

A Little Something about Asanas

The term 'asana' is sometimes mistaken as a synonym for yoga. However, that's not correct. Yoga is an eight-fold path or science of consciousness. Asanas are the third step in this eight-fold path of yoga. They are also not simply a series of movements or bodily contortions. Maharishi Patanjali defined asanas as a pose or posture that steadies the mind and body while being pleasant and comfortable. Thus, asanas must fulfil two criteria: *sthiram and sukham. Sthiram* means 'stable' and *sukham* means 'comfortable'. Only when an asana fulfils the *sthiram-sukham* criteria does it become an asana in the truest sense. Asanas are a systematically developed series of exercises intended to accentuate physical and mental training, the latter of which is more important. The primary objective of asanas is to help you achieve a healthy and supple body and a flexible yet focused mind. This is the true meaning and essence of asanas. So remember, asanas are merely a part of yoga, not synonymous with it.

Where do asanas work their magic?

Everywhere. No, really. The simplest of asanas affect every cell of your body. But if you need specifics, here it is! Asanas categorically target three sections of your body: the spine, the abdomen and your extremities. There is a final set of asanas that works on addressing the mind and body complex as a whole; those are the asanas for relaxation.

Now you would want to know how asanas affect your spine. Here's how: we find it very difficult to sit erect for a prolonged duration of time because of a stiff spine. Asanas improve the flexibility and strength of our spine. There are specific asanas that target the improvement of the spine's litheness, strength and all-around circulation i.e., forwards-bending, backwards-bending, sideways-bending and twisting.

The next section is regarding asanas and the abdomen. Most of us now have a protruding belly; this puts significant pressure on the spine as well as other abdominal organs. Various kinds of digestive issues follow. Excess belly fat also affects how we look and our self-confidence. Asanas help us get a thin waist, flat abdomen and healthy digestive organs.

A common, modern-day health issue is a constant and recurring pain in the extremities, both lower and upper. For example, many people experience joint pain in the knees, ankles, shoulders, elbows, wrists, etc. There are a number of asanas that are targeted towards improving the circulation of blood in the arms and legs, keeping joints supple, healthy and pain-free.

Asanas for relaxation help the body unwind and undergo a deep release. Often, these asanas are undervalued because rest and relaxation do not carry much importance in the modern world. However, these exercises are of vital importance for a healthy body and mind and affect creativity and productivity.

Further, asanas are not merely a physical practice. They aim to improve nervous, respiratory, digestive, circulatory and excretory systems while improving the suppleness of the body and the stability of the mind. Thus, the practice of asanas is not just physical exercise (as commonly misunderstood) but a holistic practice for overall health and vitality. This chapter has the following sections:

A. Meditative asanas for conditioning the mind, i.e., getting your mind ready
B. Sahajbhav asanas or warm up asanas for different parts of the body
C. Asanas for the spine
D. Asanas for the abdomen
E. Asanas for the extremities
F. Relaxing asanas

Now that we have understood the basics of asanas, let's know how to get started with them as well. If you want to fully uncover the potential of asana practice for your body and mind; it is important that you take a minute or two to *condition yourself*. What does this mean exactly? It means taking a minute to centre yourself and letting go of all that has been plaguing your mind. Before an asana practice, a mental cleanse or detox is of vital importance. Practising asanas with a distracted mind is not going to yield the desired benefits of holistic health. In the absence of a focused mind, an asana practice session will merely be a series of mechanical and physical motions. It is essential to condition the mind before conditioning the body. This will bring you at ease with yourself, physically and mentally. Without bodily comfort and mental equilibrium, an effective practice of asanas is not possible. Remember, *sthiram sukham* asana. Think of it as a warm-up for your mind. Here's what you need to do:

Sit in a meditative posture of your choice and focus on your breath. Choose a posture (sitting or standing) which is comfortable over a prolonged period of time. Remain in this posture for as long as you need to until you have attained that mental quietude necessary for your asana practice. Once you feel prepared, begin your asana practice.

A. Meditative Asanas for Conditioning the Mind

The specific meditative asanas for conditioning are:

1. *Sukhasana*
2. *Padmasana*
3. *Vajrasana*
4. *Stithaprarthanasana*

1. *Sukhasana*—The Easy or Pleasant Posture

I relish the feeling of peace and quietude, ensuring it extends to all activities throughout the day.

Sukhasana, as the name suggests, is a simple posture that can be maintained easily for a long time. It enables one to steady the mind and body. *Sukhasana* enables you to observe the life force. The spiritual dimension is embodied in the

term 'sukha' and 'kha' represents the wisdom of being in line
with spiritual and divine forces.

Method of Practice

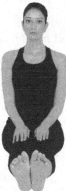

Starting Position
Sit on a mat spread on the floor with your
legs fully stretched out, without taking the
support of any wall or fixture.

Steps
1. Sit cross-legged and try to keep both
    knees a little away from the floor at an equal distance.
2. Gently place your hands on your thighs near the knees,
    palms facing downwards. There is no need for any
    hastamudra.
3. Keep your body erect, abdomen in normal contour, head
    poised and chin parallel to the ground while taking care
    not to stiffen your body. The elbows should be aligned
    with your body such that they are not pushed outwards or
    pressed inwards but are resting in a comfortable position.
4. Keep your shoulders relaxed, not drooping.
5. Sit in this position and watch
    your breath or focus on any
    object of your choice.

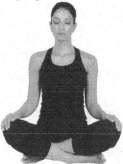

Posture Release
Straighten both your legs back
to how they were in the starting
position.

Limitations/Contraindications
- Acute arthritis.
- Psychological disorder/depression.
- There are no major limitations and can be safely practiced by anyone, with minor modifications such as sitting on a chair with one leg folded.

Benefits

Physical
- Posture gets corrected.
- It stretches your thighs, calves, ankles and hips.

Therapeutic
- It improves the flexibility of your lower extremities, especially the hip and knee joints.

Psychological
- You are more aware of your body and breathing.
- Your mind remains focused, and your concentration improves.
- This practice will make you mindful and encourage you to be in the present.
- An inner harmony arises in you, as there is less nervous agitation.

Muscles Involved
- Flexors and extensors of the vertebral column
- Abductors, flexors and medial rotators of the hip
- Knee and shoulder joint flexors

2.   *Padmasana*—The Lotus Posture

I blossom like the lotus flower, remaining unaffected by the world around me.

The word 'padma' means a lotus. The manner in which the lotus grows and blooms in full glory, unaffected by its surroundings, influences this asana. It is also a symbol of peace and is favoured by the yogis.

It is reflective of the struggles of life which you tide over to become stronger and helps you to realize that you cannot change anyone but yourself. This posture is not easy for everyone to achieve and maintain, but perseverance brings results. The formation of the body as the lotus will bring out its respective qualities within you. It ushers physical stability and psychological equanimity.

Method of Practice

Starting Position
Sit on a mat spread on the floor with your legs fully stretched out, without taking the support of any wall or fixture.

Steps
- Commence by gently bending your right leg inwards at the knee joint and fold it. With the aid of your hands, place the right heel on the top of the left thigh in such a way that the right foot is placed with its sole turned upwards.
- Likewise, place your left heel with the sole upturned over the right thigh so that the ankles cross each other. It is preferable that the ends of your heels touch closely.

- Keep both your knees pressed to the ground as far as possible.
- Hold your body comfortably erect, keeping your head, neck and trunk in a straight line. It is desirable to keep your abdomen moderately contoured inwards.
- Place your left hand just below the navel with your palm facing upwards. Place your right hand over the left hand with your palm facing upwards. Keep your shoulders and hands relaxed.
- Sit in this position, watching your breath or focus on any object of your choice.

Note: Alternate use of legs is recommended. Start by holding this pose for 1 minute and with regular practice, take it up to 10 or 15 minutes, or as per your comfort.

Posture Release
- Relax your hands and place them on your knees or thighs.
- With the help of your hands, slowly lift your top leg, place it down and relax your other leg.
- Straighten both legs slowly until you resume the starting position.

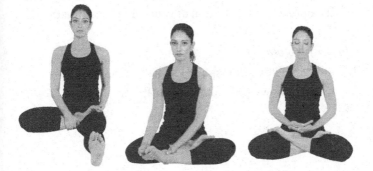

Limitations/Contraindications
- Severe arthritis and/or stiffness of the lower limbs.
- Acute knee pain.
- All limitations and contraindications of *Sukhasana* are applicable to *Padmasana* as well.

Benefits

Physical
- It stretches the thighs, calves, ankles and hips deeply.
- It corrects spinal irregularities.
- It strengthens the pelvic and lower abdomen region.

Therapeutic
- Your posture is corrected as the spine is held erect.
- Flexibility of your lower extremities improves and there is a stretch experienced in your ankle and knee joints.
- Blood circulation in your abdominal area increases.
- Helps with menstrual and sciatica issues.

Psychological
1. There is greater awareness of your body and breathing.
2. It improves concentration as your mind remains attentive.

Muscles Involved
1. Hip abductors, flexors and medial rotators.
2. Knees, elbows and ankle plantar flexors.

3. *Vajrasana*—The Adamant Posture

My strengthened body ensures a powerful mind.

This asana is inspired by the mythical weapon of immense force wielded by Lord Indra, known to have the power of a thunderbolt. It enables the development of strength of a divine nature. Symbolically, it represents spiritual prowess. *Vajrasana* is the posture that enhances strength, concentration, stability and virility.

It is the only posture that can be practised after a meal.

Method of Practice

Starting Position
Assume a kneeling position on a mat with your knees touching each other. Let your toes touch each other while the heels remain apart

Steps
- Lower yourself and sit comfortably within the hollow created by your toes and heels. If you are a beginner, use your hands to lower yourself down. You may use a soft mat.
- Keep your head and torso erect with the abdomen held in a normal contour.
- Place your hands on your knees with your palms facing downwards.
- Close your eyes and passively observe your breath or keep your gaze fixed at one point. Sit for around 5-10 minutes.

Posture Release

Slowly open your eyes and assume the starting position. Unwind your legs and gently stretch your legs forwards into a sitting position.

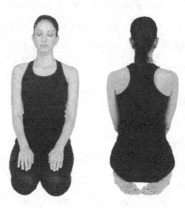

Limitations/Contraindications

- Acute arthritis.
- Very high or low blood pressure.

Benefits

Physical

- There is a correction of the posture as the spine is automatically held erect.
- It stretches the thighs, calves, ankles, hips and spine.

Therapeutic

- It improves blood circulation to the abdominal region, helping improve digestion.

- It is beneficial if you suffer from sciatica, severe lower back problems, constipation, stomach disorders, digestive problems, or acidity.
- Flexibility of the lower limbs increases.
- The generative organs get toned, along with the toning of the muscles of the hips, thighs and calves.
- It provides relief from urinary problems.

Psychological
- When practiced with open eyes this posture helps with depression as your awareness is directed at keeping your body still.
- This posture calms the mind and relaxes the nerves.
- Slow and rhythmic breathing in this position can induce a meditative state.
- Awareness of thoughts and mindfulness improves as you learn to be in the present.

Muscles Involved
- Ankle plantar flexors.
- Ankle dorsi, knee, hips and shoulder joint flexors.

4. *Sthitaprarthanasana*—The Standing Prayer Posture

The steadiness of my body is interrelated to the steadiness of my breath and mind.

A proper bearing of your body is essential for its physiological and psychological health. Faulty postural habits cause slouching and sluggishness of abdominal organs, which in turn impedes blood circulation, causing feelings of despondency, confusion, headaches, constipation, chronic fatigue, or neurasthenia (swaying of the body when you stand with your closed eyes). This pose is corrective and remedial; it boosts physical coordination and balance and promotes mental poise and spiritual elevation.

This seemingly simple posture, however, makes you acutely aware of the importance of sense faculties such as sight and breath. As in this case, you will observe that as soon as you close your eyes, the body will sway a little and you will need to manage your breath in a subtle way to steady it.

Method of Practice

Starting Position
1. Stand erect, keeping your hands at your sides and your feet together. Ensure your abdomen is held slightly inwards or in a normal contour, your pelvis tucked in gently, chest lifted slightly, but shoulders relaxed.
2. Gaze ahead, keeping your mind calm and body relaxed.

Steps
1. Fold both your hands together in the *namaskaramudra* pose and place them in front of your chest.
2. Keep your shoulders and elbows relaxed.
3. Close your eyes and observe your breath or fix your gaze at one point.
4. Stay in the position for a minimum of 5 minutes, or a maximum of 10 minutes. The aim is to hold your body motionless and not allow it to sway when your eyes are closed.

Note: In case you find you cannot maintain balance, you can stand with your feet a little apart to steady yourself or you can keep your eyes open and stare at a fixed point or place your weight on the ball of the feet near the big toes.

Posture Release
1. Slowly open your eyes and gently lower your hands to assume the starting position.
2. Maintain calmness for as long as possible.

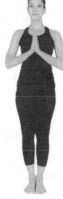

Limitations/Contraindications
- If you are suffering from acute arthritis in your lower limbs, varicose veins and hypotension, do not stand for a long time.
- In case you have vertigo, keep your eyes open with your gaze fixed and keep your feet a little apart as there is a lesser chance of toppling over.

Benefits

Physical
- It aids stance through coordination of the neuroskeletal system.
- Physical steadiness arises through control over the voluntary muscular movements.

Therapeutic
- It corrects postural defects.

Psychological
- It calms your mind and relaxes the nerves.
- Slow and rhythmic breathing in this position induces a meditative state.
- It improves concentration, as the mind remains aware.

Muscles Involved
- All postural muscles
- Elbow flexors
- Wrist extensors

Remember, it is important to allow the mind to be quiet, calm and at ease. A distracted mind is the biggest hindrance to the practice of asanas.

B. Asanas for warm-up or Sahajbhavasanas

Now that the mind is prepped, let's turn our attention towards *sahajbhavasanas*. Sahajbhavasanas are warm-up exercises that prepare the body for asana practice. The different types of Sahajbhavasanas for different muscle groups are:

1. Shayan Sahaj Bhavasan
2. Sahaj Kantha Bhavasan
3. Sahaj Bajubandhasaan
4. Sahaj Kati Madhya Bhavasan

These prevent muscle injuries. Sudden movements can cause injury; warm-up exercises help prevent sudden shocks to your body and protect the muscles, bones and joints from injury. Warm-up asanas stretch the muscles of the entire body, removing all kinds of stiffness and rigidity in the body. They also leave you feeling energized and ready for the asana practice to follow. Most, sahajbhavasanas are done standing, while some can also be done sitting. Sahajbhavasanas are meant to be performed slowly and with full awareness, just like asana practice. Breathing should also be slowly and rhythmic while practicing these postures.

So now let's know what are the various shayan sahajbhavasanas or the lying down warm up asanas and how do we do them.

1.   Shayan Sahajbhavasanas (Shsb):

In this section we will look at the following categories of warm-up asanas:
a)   *Stances For Arms, Shoulders, Hips and Legs*
b)   *Stances For the Torso*
c)   *Stances For the Torso While Lying Down*

Now we'll start with some stances for arms, shoulders, hips and legs. These practices have been specially modified for those who cannot stand or sit for any reason.

Variation 1
1.   Lie down on the floor and turn over to your right, making a pillow of your right hand and resting your head on it. Try and keep your torso erect and abdomen tucked in. The left hand should rest on the left thigh.

2. Inhaling, raise your left hand straight towards the ceiling
    and close to your head. Make a wide rotation of your
    hand and while exhaling, return to the starting position.
    Repeat twice with each hand on both sides.

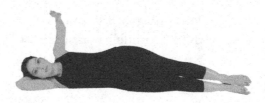

Variation 2

1. In the same starting position as above, inhale, raise your
    left hand straight towards the ceiling and swing it back to
    touch it on the floor behind.
2. As you exhale, swing your arm in an arc and touch the
    floor in the front, keeping it straight. You can also extend
    the leg behind as shown in the picture.
3. Inhale once more, raise the hand, exhale and bring it to
    rest on your thigh. Repeat on the opposite side.

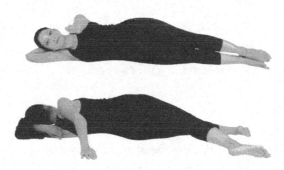

Variation 3

This variation involves a series of practices.

1. Lie straight on your back, hands flat on the ground and spread-out shoulder-level with your elbows bent. Refer to the picture shown.

2. While exhaling, bend your elbow to bring your hands down and as you inhale take the hands up. Repeat twice.

3. Next, rest your weight on your forearms. Keep your hips and legs fixed to the ground. Inhale and lift your upper body off the floor. Your head should be in contact with the floor as your chin points upwards.

4. While exhaling, lower your body down.

5. Finish off by relaxing your arms fully. Keep your legs slightly apart. Inhale and turn your feet outwards; exhale and point your feet inwards. Repeat twice.

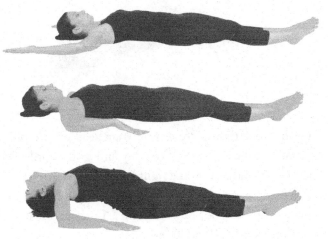

b.   Shayan Sahaj Bhav Asana Poses for the Torso

Variation 1

1. Lie on your back with your legs and feet together and hands on your sides.
2. Raise both your arms above your head to rest straight and flat on the floor, close to the ears.
3. From the waist, curve your upper body to the right as much as you can.
4. Next, curve your lower body, from the waist down, one leg at a time, beginning with moving the right leg and bringing the left leg closer to it. The body will make a 'C' formation.
5. Stay in this position for 10 or 30 seconds and try to intensify the curve, making sure that the hips do not lift off the floor.
6. Return slowly to the centre to repeat on the opposite side.

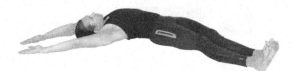

Variation 2

1. Lie on your right side, resting your head on the pillow formed by the right arm. Stretch your legs outwards; your left leg should rest on the right leg.
2. Gradually begin, pull both legs back while maintaining the same pose. The body will form a 'C' shape. Remain in this position for 10 or 30 seconds.
3. Return to the centre, turn to lie on your left side and repeat the practice.

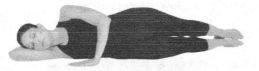

Variation 3

1. Lie on your right side, resting your head on the pillow formed by your right hand. Your left leg should be placed on your right.
1. Without moving the right leg, pull your left leg as far back as you can and remain in the position for 10 seconds.
2. Bend your left leg at the knee towards the hips and squeeze the hamstring muscles, staying there for another 10 seconds.
3. Straighten the leg, return to the centre
4. Repeat on the opposite side.

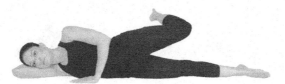

Variation 4

1. Lie on your back with your legs spread about two feet apart with arms on the sides.
2. Exhaling, contract your abdomen and hips and lift both your legs off the floor.
3. Remain in the position for 10-30 seconds, breathing normally.

4.   Inhale and relax, lowering your legs.

Variation 5

1.   Lie flat on your back.
2.   Bring the soles of both feet together, as close to the groin as possible. Use your hands to do so if necessary.
3.   Inhaling, raise both your arms above your head, stretch them and lay them flat on the ground.
4.   Remain in this position and breathe deeply from your abdominal region for 20-30 seconds.
5.   Exhaling, bring your hands to the sides and release your legs.

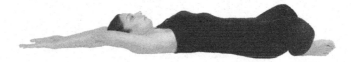

c.   Shayan Sahaj Bhavasana Poses for the torso while lying facedown

Variation 1

1.   Lie on your stomach, with your chin resting on the back of your palms placed together. Your elbows will be placed

next to your chest. Refer to the picture. Keep your legs and feet together, toes pointed.

2. Placing weight on your palms while inhaling, lift the entire abdomen off the floor.

3. Straighten your arms and look up towards the ceiling.

4. Exhale and relax your torso.

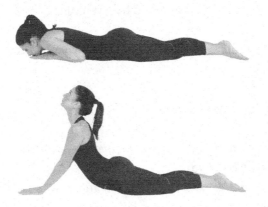

Variation 2

1. Lie on your stomach with your legs and feet together and rest your chin in your palms.

2. Inhaling, raise your right foot straight up and bend it at the knee towards the hips.

3. Exhaling, straighten your leg and lower it.

4. Repeat with the other leg.

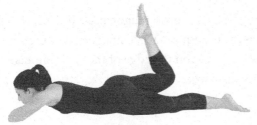

Variation 3

1. Lie on your stomach with your arms outstretched on the floor above your head and keep your legs about a foot distance apart.

2. Without lifting your hands, roll your body as much as possible to the right and then to the left. Use the strength of your core (abdomen) to help you roll.

Note: The rolling should be minimal for your hands to remain in place.

B.2 Sahaj Kantha Bhavasanas (SKB):

*This next category of warm-up asanas look at **postures for the Head and Neck (SnS)***
These exercises are excellent for those who work on a computer for long hours or have a desk job. They can be done sitting at the desk, although it is always better to stand if you can. They are the first round in a series of warm-up practices before commencing an asana session and can be done by anyone.
    Starting position for all variations:

1. Standing - Stand with your feet slightly apart or at a one-foot distance.

2. Sitting - Sit erect on a straight-backed chair without arms. In case you do not have a straight-backed chair without arms, sit firmly on the edge of the chair but take care you do not disbalance.

In all variations, remember to hold your head erect and keep your arms at your sides or on the thighs. Keep your abdomen tucked in (not constricted) and shoulders squared so that an erect posture is maintained.

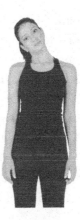

Variation 1

1. As you inhale, gently allow your head to drop towards your right shoulder without lifting your shoulder.
2. Exhaling, bring it back to the centre. Drop it to the left shoulder the same way and return to the centre.

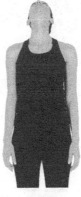

Variation 2

1. While inhaling, tilt your head backwards as far as you can without moving your shoulders or the body and gaze upwards at the ceiling.
2. While exhaling, bring your head down towards your throat, tucking your chin into the throat cavity.
3. Inhaling, return to the centre.

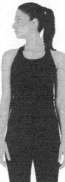

Variation 3

1. Inhale and turn your head to look on the far right and then behind. Exhale and return to the centre.
2. Repeat on the other side.

Variation 4

The following steps are done in one gentle and continuous motion.

1. Inhaling, tilt your head to the right.
2. Gently shift from the right side to the left side till you reach your left shoulder.
3. As you exhale, straighten your head till erect again. Your head should not bend forwards.
4. Repeat starting from the opposite side; go clockwise and anti-clockwise.

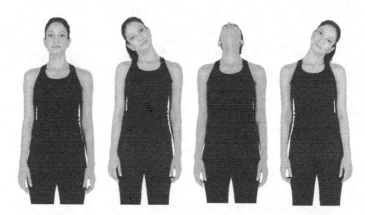

Variation 5

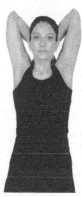

1. Clasp your hands and place them behind your head with your elbows in the front.
2. Inhaling, push your head back against your palms as they keep your head in place. Try to push the head ahead.
3. Hold for 5 seconds and relax the pressure. Repeat twice.

Variation 6

1. Place your palm on your right temple and while inhaling, push your head into the palm. Your palm must be resisting this push.
2. Exhale and relax.
3. Repeat on the opposite side.

Variation 7

1. Place your palms against your forehead and inhaling, push your head into the palms as the palms push back.
2. Exhale and relax; repeat twice.

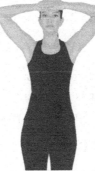

Variation 8

1. Place either one or both of your palms against your chin and inhaling, push the chin against the palm. Your palm must resist the push.
2. Exhale and relax the push; repeat twice.

Variation 9

1. Place your chin in the palms and inhaling, push the chin into the palms as the palms resist the push and press upwards.
2. Exhale and relax the push; repeat twice.

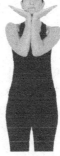

Variation 10

This variation is done standing.

1. Stand with your fingers interlaced behind you

2. Square your shoulders and push your hands and shoulders down.

3. Inhaling, look up till your chin points to the ceiling.

4. While exhaling, straighten your head and relax your shoulders. Repeat twice.

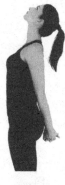

Variation 11

1. While standing or sitting, push your chin out as you inhale.

2. Exhale and relax your chin. Repeat twice.

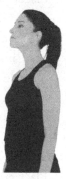

B.3 Sahaj Bajubandha Bhavasanas (SBB):

This set of warm-up asanas include postures for Shoulders, Arms, Hands and Fingers (sitting and standing)

All these practices are excellent if you work on computers for long or have a desk job. These are also a part of the warm-up practices.

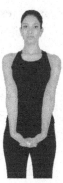

Variation 1

This posture is best done standing. In case you are sitting, spread your knees so that there is space to place your hands downwards.

1. Clasp your hands loosely clasped in the front.
2. As you inhale, push your clasped hands down as far as you can stretch them without bending forward. Keep your shoulders fixed, tucking your elbows into your waist. Stay there for 5 seconds.
3. Exhaling, relax your hands. Repeat twice.

Variation 2

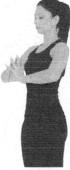

1. Place the fingertips of both your hands in front of the chest.
2. As you inhale, try to press your fingertips against each other forcefully. Hold for 5 seconds.
3. Exhaling, relax the pressure. Repeat twice.

Variation 3

Phase I

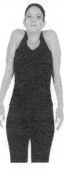

1. Keep your hands close to the sides.
2. While inhaling, lift your shoulders as high up as you can towards your ears.
3. Exhaling, relax your shoulders.
4. Repeat this motion twice.

Phase II

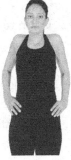

1. Place your hands on your hips and keep your head and torso erect.
2. Inhaling, extend your shoulders back, keeping the rest of your body still.
3. Exhaling, relax your shoulders. Repeat twice.

Phase III
1. Stand with hands on your sides or placed on your hips.
2. Inhaling, lift and rotate one shoulder backwards. Exhale as you bring it back to normal. Perform as a single shoulder rotation
3. Repeat with the other shoulder.

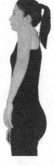

Phase IV
Practice the same with both shoulders following the same breathing rhythm.

Phase V
1. Practice shoulder rotations, rotating from the back, down and then upwards while inhaling.
2. As you exhale, bring the shoulders down.

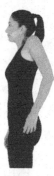

Note: You can perform this shoulder rotation with each shoulder separately too.

Variation 4
1. Clasp your hands at the back of your hips.
2. As you inhale, lift your clasped hands as high as you can from behind while keeping your shoulders down.
3. Simultaneously, lift your chin and head to look at the ceiling.
4. Exhale and relax. Repeat twice.

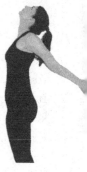

Variation 5

1. Place your fingers on your shoulders with your elbows meeting in the front.
2. As you inhale, begin the movement by raising your elbows in the front, separating and rising them upwards, going backwards and down, before returning to original form.
3. Now begin the opposite movement from the first step, while inhaling, separate your elbows and begin moving them downwards, backwards and upwards.
4. Exhaling, return to the starting position.

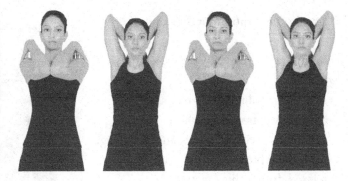

Variation 6

1. With your arms by your sides, begin lifting your right hand from the front as you inhale, raising it and bending it at the elbow to go over, behind the left shoulder.
2. Simultaneously, the left hand from below goes backwards to

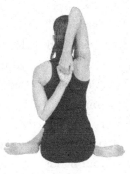

clasp the right hand. Remain in the position for 5 seconds before releasing the grasp.
3. Repeat with the opposite hands.

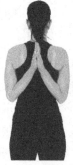

Note: You can also practice this posture seated on a chair.

Variation 7
1. Take both your hands behind from below and try to form a namaskaramudra pose at the back.
2. Stay in the position for 5 seconds.

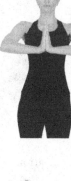

Variation 8
Phase I
*   Press your palms into a namaskaramudra a little away from your chest.
*   Inhaling, exert pressure and exhaling, release the pressure. Keep your shoulders relaxed during this practice.

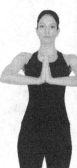

Phase II
1. Same as Phase I.
2. Press your palms together, keep your abdomen tucked in and while inhaling, raise your pressed palms together above your head.
3. Exhaling, return to the starting position. Relax the pressure and lower your hands.

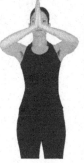

Phase III

1. Continue from Phase II, Step 2.
2. Exhaling, relax your shoulders and hands while your hands are still above your head.
3. Inhaling, press your palms and bend your elbows backwards till the fingers point downward behind the head.

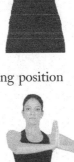

4. Exhaling, release the pressure, raise your hands with the palms still in namaskaramudra and bring them to the starting position (Step 1 of Phase I).

Phase IV

1. Start in the same position as Step 1, Phase I.
2. Pressing your palms, keep your body motionless and twist your hands to the right.
3. Return to the centre.
4. Repeat on the left side.

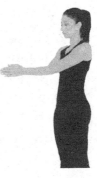

Variation 9

1. Stand with your feet a little apart and your hands raised straight in front at shoulder-level, palms together.
2. Try to join your forearms and while in this position, bend your elbows to raise the palms with your fingers pointing to the ceiling.
3. Straighten your hands. Repeat this movement three to four times.

Variation 10

Phase I

1. While inhaling, entwine your fingers at the chest and stretch out your hands.
2. While exhaling, relax the stretch.

Phase II

1. While inhaling, stretch your hands and entwine fingers as you aim your palm outwards.
2. Exhaling, relax the stretch.

Phase III

Repeat Phase I and Phase II while you take your hands up above your head.

Phase IV

Repeat Phase I and Phase II while you twist both hands to the right and then to the left.

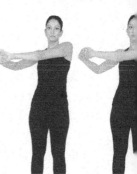

Phase V

1. Keep your hands outstretched at a shoulder-level with your right palm facing out and up.
2. While inhaling, use the left hand's fingers to push the right hand's fingers behind as much as you comfortably can.
3. Exhaling, relax. Repeat with the opposite hand.

Variation 11
Phase I
1. Stretch both your hands to shoulder-level with your palms facing down and fingers as wide apart as possible.
2. While inhaling, take your hands to the respective sides and as far back as you can without tilting your body backwards.
3. Exhaling, return to the front.

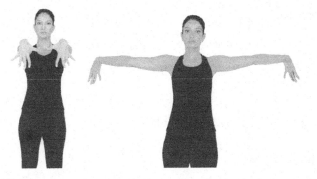

Variation 12
1. Stretch your hands out at shoulder-level and gently clench your fists.
2. Keeping the hands straight, rotate your wrists both clockwise and anti-clockwise. Repeat twice.

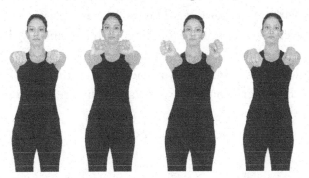

B.4 Sahaj Kati Madhya Bhavasanas (SKMB):

The final set of warm-up asanas include:

1. Torso flows
2. Postures for hips and toes,
3. Postures forFeet and toes
    3.a Standing
    3.b Sitting and
    3.c Lying Down
4. Postures for knees

1. Torso flows:

Variations for the torso include:

Variation 1 *(SnS)*
This variation can be done both standing and sitting. In this practice, the back is stretched and the abdomen is held in. If you are practising this variation while sitting, it is best done sitting on the ground with legs spread apart. In case you wish to practice sitting on a chair, sit firmly on the edge of a straight-backed chair, preferably a wooden one without upholstery. This is because plastic is too lightweight and prone to toppling. A dining chair without armrests is ideal. Keep your knees a little apart and the abdomen tucked in. Place your heels flat on the floor if you are a beginner. You can try to raise your heels with your toes on the floor.
1. Sit firmly at the edge of your chair.

2. Clasp your hands above your head, holding the head between your forearms. Keep your legs a foot apart and feet parallel to each other.

3. Inhale and tuck your abdomen in and as you exhale, in one continuous flowing movement, bend down to the right from the waist and then swing to the centre.

4. Do so again from the left side.

5. Repeat such clockwise and anti-clockwise movements twice. Ensure that during the flow, your head and hands move together.

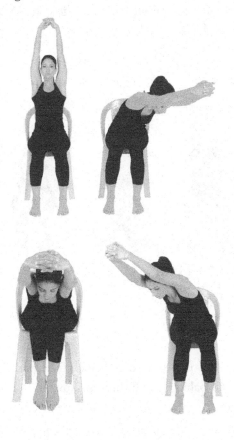

Variation 2

1. Sit firmly at the edge of your chair.
2. Inhaling, raise both your arms above your head; as you exhale, bring them down in a smooth sweep to touch your toes. In case you cannot touch your toes, go as far down as you can without disbalancing.
3. Keep your left hand fixed to your opposite foot, inhale and as you exhale, contract your abdomen, twist your torso to the right and simultaneously take your right hand up to a point towards the ceiling.
4. Look up at your raised hand and hold for 4-6 seconds; repeat on the other side.

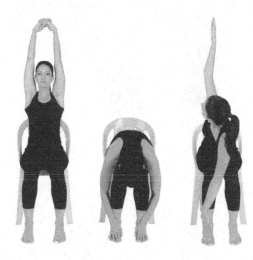

Variation 3

Phase I

1. Stand with your legs two and a half feet apart.
2. Place your palms on your hips as shown.

3. Tighten the hip muscles and as you inhale, bend backwards gently.

4. Exhaling, return to the upright position.

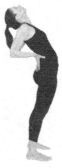

Note: Do not practice this variation if you have hypertension, cardiac ailments, or vertigo.

Hips and legs: Variations for the hips and legs generally include squats, leg lifts and lunges as they are good for the hips and legs; especially the thighs. However, in this section, new and effective practices have been described.

Variation 1

1. Stand with your legs a little apart, hands on the sides, elbows bent a little or placed on the waist.

2. Retract your right leg as though you are ready to sprint or run. The left leg will be bent. The body also will be at a slight angle; refer to the picture.

3. In this posture, the stationary leg in front will be exercised. With the body's weight on the left leg, bring the right leg forwards and upward with the knee bent and stretch it outward. In case you cannot balance, spread your hands out.

4. Hold this position with the weight on the left leg for a count of ten.

5. Extend your right leg and hold for a count of ten.

6. Bring your right foot down to the starting position.

7. Repeat with the other leg.

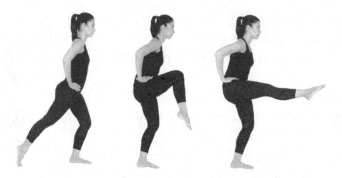

Note: In this posture, the emphasis is on the slightly bent leg with the foot on the floor, which takes on the entire body's weight.

Variation 2

1. Stand with your feet slightly apart and your hands on your hips. Throughout this variation, keep your knees slightly bent.
2. Thrust your right leg forwards and upward, keeping your toes pointed. Hold the position for a count of ten.
3. Lower your leg and pivot it upward to the right, keeping your toes pointed. Hold for a count of ten.
4. Bring the leg back to the centre.
5. Repeat all steps on the opposite side.
6. You can practice both the forwards and sideways thrust of the leg as one continuous movement once you have mastered stability on one leg.

1. Toes and feet: The toes and feet are rarely given much importance in any scheme of exercise. However, the toes and feet enable support of the body and are the aids in balanced walking. They have a number of nerve endings

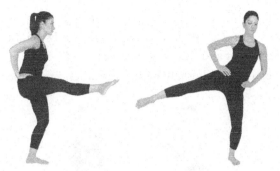

and according to reflexology, all parts of the body can be correlated to the soles of the feet. Proper care and exercise of the toes and feet is necessary.

3.a Poses for toes and feet (Standing)

Variation 1

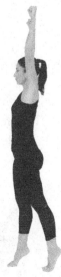

1. Raise both arms above your head and as you inhale, extend your hands to the ceiling. You can keep your fists clenched or leave your palms open. Simultaneously, raise the heels to stand on your toes.
2. Breathing normally, walk on your toes for the length of approximately 200 square feet once or twice.
3. Relax; do not overdo this practice.

3.b Poses for toes and feet (Seated Variations)

If the standing poses are too difficult for you, do these seated variations instead.

Variation 1

1. Keep your legs straight and simultaneously point the toes of one foot and flex the other set of toes.
2. Keep up this alternate movement around ten times.

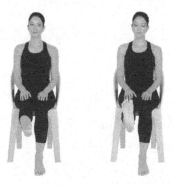

Variation 2

1. Keeping both your legs and feet together with your knees straight, rotate both feet clockwise and anti-clockwise.
2. Ensure you follow the complete movements of pointing and flexing the toes.

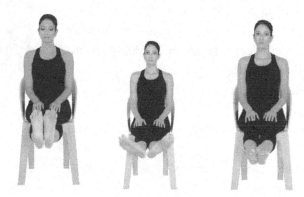

Variation 3

1. Hold the toes of one foot with all your fingers as shown.
2. Push your toes down with all your strength and at the same time, allow your fingers resist that push.

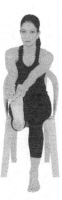

Note: You can practice with one foot at a time or both together.

Variation 4

1. Keep your legs together with your feet resting down.
2. Lift your heels off the floor. Remain in the position for 10 seconds.

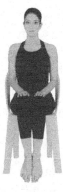

Variation 5

1. Spread your knees and feet apart; lift the heels.
2. Inhaling, raise both your hands and join the palms above your head.

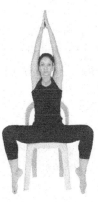

3.c Poses for toes and feet (Lying Down). These practices are excellent if, you cannot stand or sit but still want to maintain the

blood flow and flexibility of your toes and feet before you
begin your asana practice.

Variation 1
1. Lie on the floor with your feet together and your hands
    partially tucked under your hips, palms facedown.
2. Tighten your abdomen while pointing the toes and slowly
    lift both your legs off the floor as high up as you can or till
    they are at a right angle to the body.
3. Hold for 10 seconds.
4. Pointing your toes
    once more towards
    the ceiling and then
    slowly lower the legs,
    taking care that your
    lower back is well-
    supported by your hands.

Note: In case you cannot practice with both your legs together,
you can alternate the legs and raise them one at a time.

Variation 2
Follow the same steps as Variation 1, except instead of raising
your legs high, the legs are raised just about three inches off
the floor.

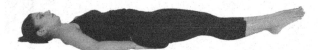

4.   Warm Up asanas for the knees.

Variation 1
1.   Lie on a mat with both your legs together and hands at the same level as your shoulders.
2.   Bend both your knees and twist your lower body so that your left knee touches the floor on the right side.

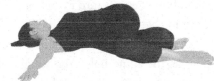

Note: You can also make movements of the knee by pressing your knee down, relaxing it and then again pressing it down.

Didn't that feel good and relaxing? Now you are ready to get to know the various asanas; let's go!

C. Asanas for the spine

Now let's begin with the spinal asanas after the warm-up asanas. The spine, known rightly as the backbone of the body, helps maintain an upright posture and supports various movements of the body such as walking, sitting, standing and even sleeping. Without a strong and supple spine, none of these movements are possible. A sedentary lifestyle contributes to a weak spine due to lack of movement, lack of awareness and an incorrect, slouchy posture. The result is back pain that can range from mild to severe or occasional to chronic.

The spine is a flexible structure, formed by a number of bones called the vertebrae that are stacked upon each other, separated by thick pads of fibrous, elastic tissues called the intervertebral discs. These discs act as shock absorbers and protect the spine from injury. There is a total of thirty-three vertebrae, with each of them having a hole in the centre. Through these holes in the vertebrae passes the spinal cord, which branches out into nerves on both sides of the spine via the joints between the vertebrae.

It is important to maintain a strong, supple and flexible spine as the spine holds the weight of your entire body and helps you to stand, sit and walk upright. It also helps to keep all your organs in place. Without a strong and well-functioning spine, it is impossible to carry out our daily functions. Modern and sedentary lifestyles further contribute to a weak and unhealthy spine as we seldom pay attention to our posture and movements, resulting in aches and pain in the spine.

Regular practice of asanas helps maintain a strong and flexible spine, improves posture and keeps the body free of aches and pains. Asanas that focus on complete spinal circulation are the most effective as they ensure that the spine remains flexible and strong. Mindful movements in coordination with your breath further helps avoid unwanted injury to the spine and this is where the practice of asanas with a Yogendra rhythm becomes important.

Asanas for the spine

1. Parvatasana (all variations)
2. Talasana (all variations)
3. Konasana I and II
4. Vakrasana (all variations)

5. Bhujangasana

1. *Parvatasana*

The Mountain Posture
Being steady and firm strengthens both my mind and body.

The mountain posture reflects the ideals of stability, steadfastness and resoluteness. This posture has three variations to provide the spine with different kinds of stretches and movements—upwards, backwards, forwards, sideways and a twist)—while maintaining a firm base stance. It also makes us aware of the importance of the faculty of sight, which needs to be focused to allow us to maintain balance. In case you cannot sit on the floor, practice standing or sitting on a chair without arm support.

Method of Practice

Starting Position
1. Sit erect in padmasana or sukhasana and keep your hands at their respective sides, palms facing upwards. Keep your head and neck straight and your abdomen tucked in gently.
2. Keep your eyes focused on a single point ahead.

Steps
1. Inhaling, raise both your arms together from the sides for an upward stretch, joining the palms to each other overhead
2. Keep your arms close to the respective ears, your abdomen gently pulled inwards and your back straight. Avoid

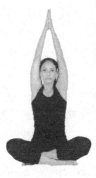

bending your arms at the elbows and wrists and keep them stretched and straight.

3. Fix your gaze fixed on a single point ahead.

4. Maintain this position for 6 seconds, retaining your breath.

Posture Release

While exhaling, turn your palm outwards and lower your arms while still extended to the sides.

Variation 1

Starting Position

In the starting position described above, raise both your arms together from the sides to join your palms overhead, keeping the arms straight and close to your ears.

Steps

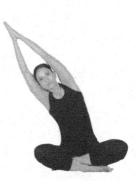

1. While inhaling, bend to the right side while keeping your hips firmly on the floor; your head tucked in between the arms. There should be no movement below the waist.

2. Immediately exhaling, return to the centre.

3. Inhaling, bend towards the left side.

4. Immediately exhaling, return to the centre.

5. Turn the palms outwards and while exhaling, bring them
    down to the respective sides to touch the floor.

Variation 2
Starting Position
Follow the same steps till Step 3 of Variation 1.

Steps
1. While exhaling, twist your spine, pivoting towards the
    right side, maintaining stillness below the waist. This is
    an axial movement; maintain the head,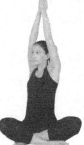
    hands and upper torso as one unit
    while twisting.
2. Immediately return to the central
    position while inhaling.
3. Exhaling, twist towards your left side.
4. Inhaling, return to the central position.

Variation 3
Starting Position
Same as Variation 1.

Steps
1. Inhaling, bend backwards a little so that your spine arches
    backwards and keep the head locked in between your
    arms. Look upwards and backwards while maintaining
    the base stance. Note that this does not involve too much
    backward bending.
2. Now, while exhaling, bend forwards so that your upper
    body is parallel to the floor; keep your head locked

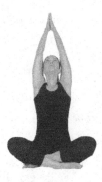

in between the arms and move harmoniously. You will notice a compression in your abdomen.

3. Maintain this position and suspend your breath for 6 seconds.
4. Inhaling, return to the centre.
5. As you exhale once more, bring your hands down to the sides.

Note: You can perform these variations as a series and once you have finished, return to the starting position with your hands down by the side.

Limitations/Contraindications
1. Arthritis of the knees and frozen shoulders.
2. Those who cannot sit on the ground, although you can practice while sitting in a straight-backed chair.
3. Hypertension and cardiac patients must not hold their breath and avoid variations.

Benefits

Physical
1. It stretches all your abdominal and pelvic muscles and loosens your hip joints.
2. It exercises your inactive waist zone and helps reduce a flabby abdomen.

Therapeutic
1. It corrects minor postural defects of the spine and stretches the muscles of your back.

2. Unnatural curvature of the spine and minor displacements of the vertebrae are corrected.
3. Internal organs in your abdominal region get an internal massage; there is improved blood circulation.

Psychological
1. It improves the ability to stay focused.
2. It develops strength, stability and longevity.
3. The mind gains a deeper understanding of strength from the body.

Muscles Involved
- Hip abductors, flexors and medial rotators.
- Extensors of the vertebral column.
- Shoulder flexors.

2. *Talasana – The Palm Tree Posture*

I lift myself up, committing to being unswayed by the tides of the world.

This form of this asana and the movement involved is based on the palm tree. The immense flexibility and stability is the quality that needs to be developed within us—physically as well as psychologically—through the practice of this asana. This posture stretches the muscles of the body. It has four variations.

Variation 1
Starting Position
- Stand erect with your hands at your sides, shoulders relaxed but squared, chest lightly expanded and abdomen

held firm but in a normal contour. Keep your feet parallel
to each other maintaining a foot between them.

- Avoid a forwards or backward stance. Focus your eyes at
  one point straight ahead.

Steps

- While inhaling, raise your right arm forwards
  and up towards the ceiling, rising on the toes
  in a synchronized manner.

- Retain the position and hold your breath for
  6 seconds.

- The right arm must remain close to your ear
  in the final seconds. The other arm is straight
  and relaxed by the side. Ensure both your
  arms are straight, but not stiff.

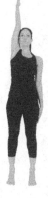

Posture Release

Turn your palm to face outward and while exhaling, keeping
your arm straight, lower it through a backward and downward
rotational movement. Simultaneously, lower the heels to assume
the starting position. Repeat the steps with your left hand.

Note: During the completion of this movement, your hand
must reach the side of your thigh and your feet must touch
down at the same time.

Variation 2

Maintain the same technique, except instead of alternating
hands, raise both your hands at the same time and bring them
back down together in a similar manner.

Variation 3
The same technique is followed, except you raise both your arms simultaneously from the sides, palms facing outwards and the posture culminates when the two palms meet overhead. Return to the starting position in the same way as mentioned earlier.

Variation 4
With the technique remaining the same, cross both your hands at the wrists in front of your body as a starting point. Then, raise your crossed hands above your head while inhaling. Return to a similar manner as stated before.

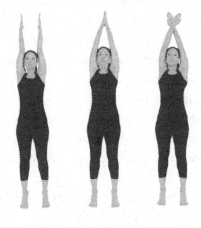

Limitations/Contraindications
- Spinal injury and abnormalities.
- Frozen shoulder and arthritis.
- Hypertension and serious cardiac complaints.
- Muscular and nervous agitation.

Benefits

Physical
- It facilitates the maximum stretching of your body.
- It enables free and natural accommodation for the internal organs.
- Coordination of muscular activity improves.
- It tones the usually relaxed muscles of your abdomen.

Therapeutic
- It develops the respiratory muscles and their vital indexes.
- There is a thorough expansion of the lungs due to the movements of the upper body.
- Flexibility of the spinal column improves and due to the stretch on the vertebral column, undue pressure on the vertebrae is released.
- By stretching the ankles and shoulder joints, problems of stiffness stemming from arthritis can be reduced.
- It improves reflexes and neuromuscular coordination.
- It tones the muscles of your legs and improves the venous function.
- It improves the balance of the body and the gait.
- It relieves sciatica pain and flat feet.

Psychological
- It helps maintain a balanced state of mind.
- It helps in remaining unaffected by the rhythms of the world.

Muscles Involved
- Planter flexors of the ankle, extensors of the vertebral column and the shoulder flexors
- Hip abductors and abductors as stabilizers
- Shoulder extensors are exercised when reversing

3. *Konasana I and II - The Angle Posture*

Kona means 'angle'. The body takes the form of an angle in this asana. In this posture, there are three variations taking the body through different motions. In forming angles, your body is bent and twisted in ways not normally used in day-to-day activities. Most of the bending and twisting in konasana is from the waist, which results in streamlining the contours of your abdomen. There is an internal massage of the organs of the stomach through compression.

There are three variations of this posture at The Yoga Institute and they are explained below.

Variation 1
Adjustments and compromises are two sides of the same coin, inhibiting rigidity and stimulating the flexibility of the body and mind.

Starting Position
1. Stand with your feet parallel, around three feet apart and keep your hands on the sides.
2. Turn your head to face the right.
3. Rest your left palm lightly on the waist, palm facing down (at a right angle to the body), the fingers in the front and thumb behind.

Steps

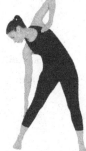

1. While inhaling, as you bend laterally from the waist to the right side, let your right hand glide down as far as it can go.

2. Simultaneously, allow your left hand at the waist to slide up towards the armpit.

3. Maintain this posture as you hold your breath for 6 seconds and ensure that your body, arms and elbows are not tilting forwards or backwards. In this position, your gaze is fixed on the fingers of your right hand.

Posture Release

1. Exhaling, return to the starting position by letting your left-hand glide down while straightening your body.

2. Allow your right hand to glide to your waist to repeat the same process on the opposite side.

3. Let both your hands down to the side. Bring your feet together or leave them apart if you are practicing more rounds of this asana or its variations.

Note: Keep your hips and legs fixed as you bend sideways.

Variation 2
To be like the blade of grass, bending, if need be, but not too much; recognizing the importance of my spiritual self.

Starting Position
Stand with your feet parallel around three feet apart. Keep your hands on the sides.

Steps
1. Raise your left hand from the side, held straight with the palm facing out so that your arm is close to the ear while your right hand loosely hangs by your side.

    You should be facing ahead.
2. While inhaling, bend from the waist laterally to the right as far as you can go without tilting to the front or back.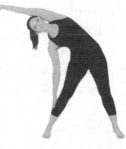
3. Maintain this position while holding your breath for 6 seconds.

Posture Release
1. While exhaling, return to the starting position and lower your left hand.
2. Repeat on the opposite side.
3. On completion of bending on both sides, let your hands hang loosely at the sides and bring your feet together or leave them apart if you are practicing more rounds of this asana or its variations.

Variations for Konasana I have designed:
Sitting Variations: These include three variations.

Variation 1

Practice 1

1. Sit erect in sukhasana, keeping your abdomen tucked in with both your hands on the floor beside your hips.
2. Raise your right hand from the side and bring your arm close to the ears.
3. Inhaling, bend your torso to the left. Remain in the position for 6 seconds while retaining your breath.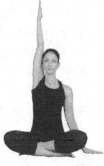
4. Exhaling, return to the original position.
5. Repeat on the opposite side with the opposite hand.

Practice 2

1. Follow till Step 2 as outlined in the previous practice.
2. Inhale as you stretch your hand upwards; exhale as you twist your torso slightly to the left and bend.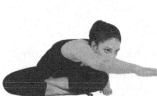
3. Inhaling, return to the centre.
4. Repeat on the opposite side with the opposite hand.

Practice 3

1. Sitting erect with your legs apart and abdomen tucked in, clasp both hands behind your head.

2. Inhale and as you exhale, bend your torso to the right, contracting your abdomen.

3. Inhaling, return to the centre and exhaling, bend to the opposite side.

4. Inhaling, return to the centre.

5. Repeat three to five times on both sides.

Variation 2

1. Sit in padmasana.

2. Repeat all the above movements as described in practice 1, 2 and 3 described above while sitting in padmasana.

Lying Down Variations: These include two variations.

Variation 1

1. Lie on your back on a mat with your arms on the sides.

2. Raise both your hands, sliding them along the floor, till your arms are touching the ears straight above your head.

3. Bend your upper body along with the arms towards the right side as much as you can.

4. Now, take your right leg, gliding it on the floor as far to the right as you can.

5. Let your left leg follow the right leg as closely as you can.

6. Check that your entire body is touching the ground. It would have formed a C-shaped curve.

7. Stay in this position for at least 30 seconds to a minute, pointing and flexing your toes alternately.

8. Slowly return to the centre and repeat on the opposite side.

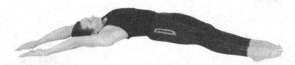

Variation 2

1. Repeat steps 1 to 4 of the asana described above.
2. Slide your left leg in the opposite direction (to the right).
3. Stay in the position for 30 seconds to a minute.
4. Return to the centre and repeat on the opposite side.

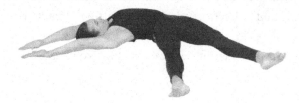

4. *Vakrasana – The Curve Posture*

I become self-aware and ever vigilant, especially during the unexpected turns and twists of life.

Vakra means 'curve'. The formations and the process of this asana involve curving the torso to twist to the spine. It can be done sitting, standing, or lying down. It is useful for those who have a desk job. The waist and the abdominal organs get exercised.

Sitting

Starting Position
1. Sit on a mat with your legs fully stretched forwards, toes pointing upwards and your hands beside your body with the palms resting on the mat.
2. Keep your back straight; neck and head in line.
3. Stretch both your hands forwards and raise them to shoulder-level. Keep your palms facing downwards. Inhale.

Steps
1. Exhaling, twist your spine towards the right as much as you can while ensuring that your head, neck, shoulders, hands and the torso move as one unit.
2. Keep the hands parallel to each other and keep your lower body firmly fixed to the ground.
3. Immediately, while inhaling, come to the centre.
4. Exhaling, twist towards your left side in the same manner.
5. Return to the centre while inhaling.

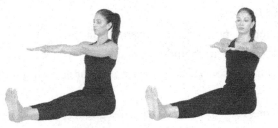

Posture Release
While exhaling, put your hands down to the sides of your thighs.

Limitations/Contraindications
- Severe back pain.
- Abdominal inflammations, ulcers and hernia.
- Sciatica.

Benefits

Physical
- It relaxes the muscles of your back
- It strengthens the muscles of your lower back.
- It exercises your abdominal muscles.

Therapeutic
- Low back pain is alleviated.
- Flab on the lateral side of the abdomen gets reduced.
- It relieves stiffness of the vertebrae.

Psychological
It increases concentration, making you alert and attentive.

Muscles Involved
- Lateral rotators of the vertebral column.
- Flexors of the shoulder joints.
- Isometric contractions of the anterior abdominal wall.

Variations for Vakrasana I have designed:

Variation 1
1. Stand with your legs roughly two feet apart.

2. While inhaling, raise your hands from the front to the level of your shoulder.

3. While exhaling, twist your torso to the right as far as you can, while simultaneously stretching the right hand as far behind as possible.

4. The left-hand bends at the elbow. Refer to the picture.

5. Take care not to raise your left foot during this extreme twist and avoid turning your left hip or thigh.

6. Remain in the position for 6 seconds.

7. While inhaling, return to the centre.

8. As you exhale, repeat the same on the left side.

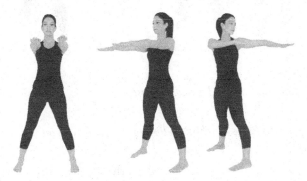

Variation 2

1. Repeat Step 1 of Variation 1.

2. Raise your hands to shoulder-level and clasp your fingers.

3. Bend your torso, putting your head between your arms and continue bending, but keep the body straight to form a right angle at the hip. Your hands should be stretched straight out.

4. Contract the abdomen and while exhaling, turn your torso from the hip to the right.

5. Remain like this for 6 seconds.
6. While inhaling, return to the centre but do not rise.
7. As you exhale, repeat on the opposite side.
8. While inhaling, return to the centre, straighten up, release
    your hands and bring them to the sides.

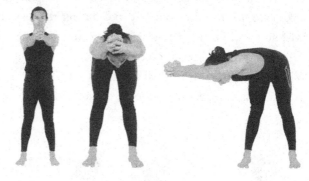

5. *Bhujangasana – The Cobra Posture*

*All potentials lie within; believing this, I rely on my inner
strengths.*

The way the head is raised in the final position in this
asana is similar to a fanned cobra and hence, the name. The
purpose of creating this posture is to imbibe the qualities
observed in a cobra: determination, alertness and precision,
all of which are most desirable qualities for a *sadhaka* on the
path of yoga.

This is a backwards-bending asana.

Method of Practice

Starting Position
Lie down on a mat, flat on your stomach with your hands at the sides of your body.

Steps
1. Bending at the elbows, place your palms facedown near your chest, keeping your elbows close to your body.
2. Inhaling, raise your head and neck upwards to look up at the ceiling.
3. Raise your upper body only until the navel, not more and make sure that your feet remain together.
4. Remain in the final position, holding your breath for 6 seconds.

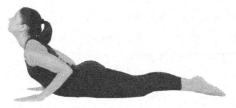

Posture Release
Exhaling, bring your head, neck and torso down to rest on the mat.

Limitations / Contraindications
- Hypertension, heart ailments
- Pregnancy, peptic ulcers, hernia
- Hyperthyroid

Benefits

Physical

- It tones the deep muscles that support the spinal column and trunk.
- There is stimulation of the spinal nerves.
- It massages and stimulates the adrenal gland.
- It tones the abdominal muscles.

Therapeutic

- The alternate contractions and subsequent relaxation corrects minor displacements of vertebra.
- It reduces constipation and flatulence.
- It relieves generalized muscular pain.

Psychological

It helps develop faith and self-confidence.
    It develops a calm state of mind.
    It strengthens willpower.

Muscles Involved

Sternomastoid and pectoralis major.
    Extensors of the vertebral column and neck.
    Isometric contraction of the muscles of the upper limbs.

My Variation of *Bhujangasana:*

Variation 1
1. Lie on your stomach with your legs together.

2. Your hands are placed with your palms facedown near your chest.

3. While inhaling, raise your entire torso off the floor with the head tilted backwards, looking up.

4. Your back should be arched and the hands straightened.

5. Remain in this position for 6 seconds.

6. While exhaling, return to the starting position.

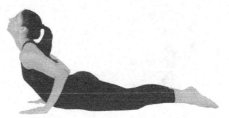

Variation 2

1. Lie on your stomach with your legs together.

2. Your hands should be clenched behind.

3. While inhaling, raise your torso off the floor with your head tilted backwards, looking up.

4. Your back will be arched and the hands straightened.

5. Remain in this position for 6 seconds.

6. While exhaling, return to the starting position.

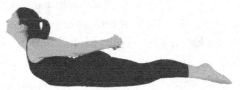

Variation 3
1. Lie on your stomach with your legs slightly apart.
2. Place your hands on the floor as in the original posture.
3. While inhaling, raise your entire body off the floor.
4. Remain in this position for 6 seconds.
5. While exhaling, return to the starting position.

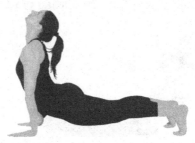

D. Asanas for the abdomen

The objective of asana practice is to foster harmony between the body and mind and ensure smooth functioning and synchronisation of both. The abdominal region of the body is one of the most important regions since it is where all your digestive organs are located. It is the energy-giving region as food is digested, assimilated and excreted from here. Hence, it is vital that the abdominal region is always strong and healthy. Most diseases arise because of an unhealthy gut; keeping the abdominal organs healthy is of utmost importance.

Other than keeping the organs healthy and the abdominal region strong, our emotions also affect this area. It is important to open up this region to let go of negative and unhealthy emotions from our system. Most of our physical and mental health depends on the health of the abdominal region.

It is essential to strengthen the muscles of the abdominal region, keep the organs healthy and improve blood circulation in this region. There are various kinds of asanas that include compression and stretching of the abdominal region. Practising these asanas correctly helps improve the tone of the muscles, as well as the organs in the abdominal region. It also enriches and enhances blood circulation, resulting in better digestion and healthier organs.

The Abdominal Asanas

1. Konasana III
2. Yoga mudra
3. Pavan muktasana (All variations)
4. Yogendra chakrasana
5. Paschimottasana

How to do them?

1. Konasana III

The Angle Posture

Variation 3
I spread myself unto the universe, twisting and bending in the melee, recognizing my potential to accomplish the goal.

This variation of the angle pose constitutes multiple actions. It involves lateral twisting and forwards bending of your spine. It creates abdominal compression and an extension to the spine during the twisting and bending.

Starting Position

1. Stand with your feet, 2.5 feet distance apart, hands at your side, feet parallel to each other.

Steps

1. Raise both your hands from the front, palms facing upwards till the shoulder-level.
2. Inhaling, spread your hands to the respective sides and turn the head to the right (the hands are still spread apart). Fix your gaze on the fingers of your right palm and follow the palm as it moves.
3. Exhaling, twist your upper body from the waist towards the left and bend down so that your right hand touches the left toe. The head is bent down. Your left hand swings straight upwards towards the ceiling
4. Twist your head and neck to take the gaze up to look at the left hand. Hold this position for 6 seconds with suspension of breath.
5. Now look down and again fix your gaze on the right palm.
6. Inhaling, bring your body up straight continuing to look at the right palm till you are standing straight. The hands are spread apart. Exhale.
7. Now turn your head to the left, practice all the steps on the opposite side.
8. Once you have come up, exhaling, bring your hands down to the respective sides. Relax by bringing your feet together.

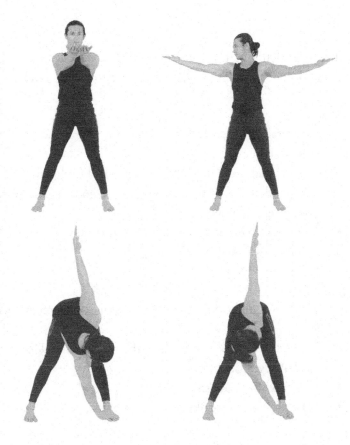

Limitations / Contraindications

- Hypertension, severe cardiac problems
- Vertigo
- Facet joint abnormalities, scoliosis, resolving and acute disc prolapse, osteoarthritic spinal problems
- Hernia, abdominal surgeries

Benefits

Though each variation of Konasana has its own intrinsic benefits, all have multiple benefits on the following levels.

Physical
- It stretches, massages and tones the lateral muscles of your waist.
- Your shoulder and hamstring muscles get healthy stretches.
- Intra-abdominal compression gives a good massage to your internal organs.
- It improves your abdominal muscle tone.
- It increases flexibility of your spine.

Therapeutic
- There is a mild readjustment of the spine and strengthens a weak spine.
- It is good for muscular pains of the cervical, shoulder and lumbar regions.
- It is good for scoliosis.
- It helps managing ankylosing spondylitis.

Psychological
- The physical benefits have effects on your mind at a very subtle level.
- It brings peace to your mind as your body is relaxed at the physical level.
- It brings attention inwards creating awareness of the physical self.
- It improves the synchronization between your mind and body.

Muscles Involved
- Sternomastoid
- Erector spinae
- Serratus anterior and trapezius
- Anterior shoulder and lateral trunk
- Hip abductors and gluteus maximus

2. Yoga Mudra

Vairagya: letting go is as essential as the breath exhaled.

Yoga Mudra symbolizes yoga. It polarizes the opposites. It brings about humility in the presence of achievement. It is representative of grace and modesty within greatness. It is the emblem of great understanding and wisdom which knows the frailty of human nature and also its boundless potential.

Method of Practice

Starting Position
1. Sit in padmasana or sukhasana, clasp your hands behind your back; the right hand holding the wrist of the left hand. Keep your head, neck and torso comfortably erect.
2. Focus your gaze at one point ahead of you or close your eyes.

Steps
1. While exhaling, bend forwards to touch your forehead to the ground.
2. Maintain the position, suspending your breath for 6 seconds.
3. While inhaling, raise your torso to the sitting position.

4. While exhaling, bend your torso to the right to touch your forehead to your right knee.
5. While inhaling, return to the centre.
6. While exhaling, repeat on the left side.
7. Inhaling, rise and return to the centre.

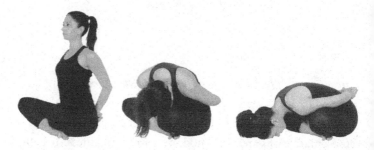

Posture Release

Exhaling, release the hands and bring them to the front to rest them on the knees.

Notes:

- While bending forwards to touch your forehead to the floor or your knees, make sure that the hips do not rise and that the lower body is firmly fixed to the ground.

- In case you are unable to touch your forehead to the floor, let your knees go down as far as possible without the hips being lifted.

- Ensure that your shoulders remain relaxed when the forehead touches the floor or the knees.

- You can practice this asana in a static way by remaining in the final position with the forehead touching the floor in front for a minute or two.

Limitations/Contraindications

- Hypertension, cardiac ailments.
- Hernia, abdominal surgery.
- Cervical and lumbar spondylitis.
- High myopia, glaucoma, serious eye disorders.
- Acute pain in the neck and back, stiffness of the back and joints.

Benefits

Physical

- There is stretching of almost all the posterior muscles of the trunk and the neck.
- It improves muscle tone.
- Deep intra-abdominal compression affects the viscera favourably.

Therapeutic

- The lateral stretch stimulates vital areas of the colon. The ascending and descending colon gets good pressure, alleviating constipation.
- Acceleration of the venous flow from the sex organs improves favourably.
- The compression of the diaphragm and the abdominal walls provides a massage to the abdominal organs and is useful in gastric conditions.
- It helps prevent sagging of the uterus and postnatal laxity.
- Lumbar pain is alleviated.
- Improves the overall health of the abdomen and pelvic organs due to good blood circulation and drainage.

- There is a favourable change in the management of ankylosing spondylitis.

Psychological
- It helps to soothe and calm the mind.
- It brings fosters a sense of humility and gratitude.

Muscles Involved
- Extensors of the vertebral column
- Hip abductors, flexors and medial rotators
- Knee flexors
- Shoulder girdle retractors

3. Pavanamuktasana—The Air Free Posture

Not holding on to things; I 'let go' and feel relief, both emotionally and physically.

Our body accumulates stresses of all kinds. When they are released, there is a wave of peace and relaxation. This asana is very simple to perform yet has plenty of benefits. The practice of this posture releases flatulence and helps relieve indigestion and constipation. You can enjoy the benefits of this asana by performing in a dynamic way or you can remain in the posture for 1-2 minutes while breathing normally.

Note: Those with a weak abdomen or those not used to exercise are requested not to put pressure in the final position.

Variation 1—Ekapada (with one leg)

Starting Position

1. Lie supine on a mat with your feet together and hands at the sides and inhale.

Steps

1. Exhaling, raise your right leg, fold it at the knee joint and clasp your knee (or shin) with both your hands interlocking at the arms.
2. Pull the knee up to your chest and keep it firmly pressed, suspending your breath.
3. Maintain the posture for 6 seconds.

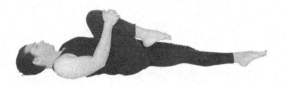

Posture Release

1. Release your clasped hands, inhale, straighten your leg and bring it to the starting position.
2. Repeat with the other leg.

Variation 2—Dvipada (with both legs together)

The steps are the same as before except you must perform them by lifting both legs together.

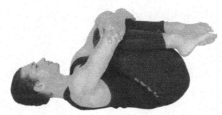

Limitations/Contraindications
- Abdominal surgery, inflammation, pain.
- Cardiac ailments.
- Hernia, piles.
- Not recommended for women during menstruation and pregnancy.

Benefits

Physical
- It stretches your lower back, hips and thighs.
- The intra-abdominal compression provides good circulation and massages your abdomen and pelvic viscera.
- It stretches your arms, shoulders and neck.

Therapeutic
- This posture offers flatulence relief by quickening the movement and expulsion of the intestinal flatus.
- A flabby abdomen, subnormal functions of the abdominal viscera and pelvic organs respond favourably to this posture.

- There is a deep internal pressure massage and stretching of the networks of muscles, ligaments and tendons of the waist zone and the pelvis.
- It aids in resolving chronic constipation, sluggish liver, weak functioning of the abdominal and the pelvic organs.

Psychological
- It alleviates mental sluggishness by enabling the release of toxins from the body.
- It brings about mental clarity.

Muscles Involved
- Hip, knee, finger flexors
- Shoulder muscles, triceps, gluteus maximus and hamstrings

My Variations:

Variation 1—Standing
1. Stand with your feet together and hands on the sides.
2. Lift your right leg, bending it at the knee and with both your hands, press the knee into your abdomen.
3. Hold the position for a few seconds and lower your leg.
4. Repeat with the other leg.

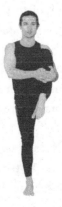

Variation 2—Sitting

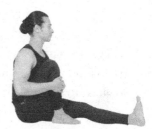

1. Sit with both your legs outstretched and together.
2. Bend your right leg at the knee and press the knee into your stomach using both hands.
3. Release your right leg and repeat with your left leg.
4. You can practice the pose with both your legs drawn towards your stomach and your knees clasped within your arms.

4. Yogendra chakrasana—The Wheel Posture

Like the wheel in constant motion, I move ahead, breaking free from the past.

Chakrasana represents the wheel. The wheel is a primary invention in the world and has enabled endless functions. Its movement generates energy. It is a fundamental part of history! Chakrasana is performed in four phases. It is recommended you practice the steps before you can practice the entire four phases seamlessly and then incorporate the breathing rhythms. You can also break up the practices and master each phase and related breathing rhythms. Later, practice them all together.

Note: The steps of this asana are slightly complicated. It is best to try all the steps and phases independently before you integrate the breathing rhythms.

Method of Practice

Starting Position
1. Stand with your feet around two feet apart with your hands at the sides.

Steps—Phase I
1. Clench your fists and while inhaling, raise your hands above the head. Your arms must be held straight and close to your ears; this and the second step must flow seamlessly.
2. Arch your back as much as possible and look up without tilting your hips and waist forwards. The body below your waist remains fixed.
3. This step will have to be mastered before the breathing rhythm is incorporated.

Steps—Phase II
1. As you exhale, bring your hands and head down together towards the feet in a sweeping arc; refer to the picture.
2. Lower your head as close to the knees as possible.

Steps—Phase III
1. In a sweeping motion, take your arms behind your back as high up as you can.

Steps—Phase IV
1. Clasping your hands at the back, take your head further towards the knee, forming a full circle.
2. Perform all the steps from Phases III to IV are as you exhale.

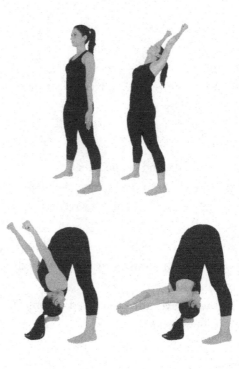

Posture Release

1. While inhaling, unclasp your hands, clench your fists and with your head still lowered, bring your hands down.
2. Holding the head in between your arms, raise your torso to the Phase I position.
3. Lower your hands as you exhale.

Limitations / Contraindications

*   High blood pressure.
*   Cardiac problems.
*   Hernia, piles.
*   Abdominal inflammation.

- High myopia, glaucoma, serious eye disorders.
- Spinal injuries.

Benefits

Physical
- It strengthens the muscles of your chest and waist.
- It develops the muscles of your back, neck, spine and shoulders.
- It strengthens the core.
- It exercises the anterior and posterior muscles of your body.

Therapeutic
- It acts as a remedial and preventive measure for constipation.

Psychological
- It improves the balance of your mind.
- It brings fosters a sense of humility and gratitude.

Muscles Involved
- Retraction of the scapula.
- Extensors, abductors and internal rotators of the shoulder.
- Posterior trunk muscles and the gluteus maximus.

My Variation for Chakrasana

Method of Practice
1. Lie on your back on a mat and bend your knees, keeping your legs together.

2. Take your hands above your head, bending them at the elbows to place your palms flat on the ground a little away from the head.

3. Taking support of your hands (the body weight shifts to your hands) as you inhale, lift the torso off the floor as high up as possible.

4. While exhaling, slowly lower your body.

5. Bring your hands to the starting position.

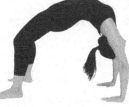

5. Paschimottasana—The Posterior Stretch

Self-effort takes me to a point. It is self-offering that makes me strong.
The word 'paschim' means west and is used in the context of the posterior of the body and *uttana* for stretching. The need for spinal fitness is obvious. Exercising it in all possible ways is essential. Paschimottasana builds a strong and healthy spine, which in turn upholds the body. However, it is the intense abdominal compression that strengthens the core. The process of the practice of this asana and its final form brings about a sense of achievement devoid of ego and cultivates humility. You can perform this asana in a dynamic way as mentioned below or you can remain in the final posture for 1-2 minutes breathing normally.

Method of Practice

Starting Position
1. Sit on a mat with your legs fully stretched and your toes pointing upwards.

2. Keep your spine, shoulders, neck erect and look straight ahead.

3. Keep your hands relaxed beside your body with your palms facedown.

Steps

1. While inhaling, lean backwards and keep both your hands beside your chest folded at the elbow, palms facedown. Your elbows should not jut out.

2. While exhaling, bend forwards and stretch your hands out to hold the toes.

3. Try to touch the head to the knees without bending your knees. At this stage, you could try lowering your elbows to touch the floor if possible.

Posture Release

1. Remain in the posture for 6 seconds with your breath suspended.

2. While inhaling, return to the starting position.

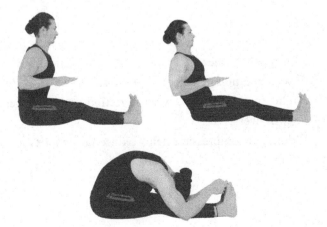

Caution: This final position is not easily attained. It is recommended that you try as much as you can and practice regularly. Overdoing this practice may cause injury.

Limitations/Contraindications
- Hypertension, heart ailments.
- Pregnancy, peptic ulcers, hernia.
- Hyperthyroid.
- Serious spinal disorders.
- Myopia, glaucoma and serious eye disorders.

Benefits

Physical
- It causes deep intra-abdominal compressions and massages your abdominal viscera.
- It stretches the superficial and deep muscles of your ankles, legs and shoulders.
- It stretches the spine and improves flexibility.

Therapeutic
- A deep posterior stretch to the spine helps corrects minor deformities in the curvature of the spine and improves blood circulation in veins and arteries.
- It relieves constipation, weak digestion and improves a sluggish liver.
- Abdominal compression helps reduce fat deposits in the abdomen.

Psychological
- It acts as a stress reliever.
- It calms your mind.
- It enhances your concentration.

Muscles Involved
- Ankle dorsi, knee, shoulder, finger and plantar flexors
- Vertebral column, hip and knee extensors
- Isometric contraction of forearm, arm, shoulder girdle
- Abductor, medial rotators

My Variation for Paschimottasana

Method of Practice
1. Steps 1 to 4 remain the same as in the main practice.
2. While exhaling, turn your torso to the right as far as possible and lean forwards.
3. Extending your hands, try to touch the floor ahead on the right and ensure that your left hip does not lift.
4. Remain in the position for 6 seconds.
5. Inhaling, return to the centre.
6. While exhaling, repeat on the opposite side.
7. Inhaling, return to the centre.
8. Exhaling, lower hands and relax your hands on the thighs.

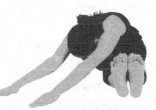

E. Asana for the extremities

Aches and pain in the extremities have become common problems these days. The human body has two extremities: upper and lower. Your upper extremities are your hands and the lower extremities are your legs. Pain in the joints and muscles of extremities is caused primarily due to stiffness and a lack of proper blood circulation. It is crucial to ensure the sufficient movement and stretching of the extremities. Asanas that strengthen extremities help increase lubrication of the joints and strengthen the muscles. This will ensure that stiffness and tension are relieved, reducing pain to a significant extent.

Regular and consistent practice contributes to the strengthening and toning of muscles in the extremities. Asanas that target extremities are extremely beneficial for athletes like runners or badminton players. It is also beneficial for office workers who are constantly sitting in one place. Along with postural issues, joints and muscle aches are also very common for this group. Since yoga aims to be preventive in nature, practice of these asanas will help to avert severe arthritis and other ailments pertaining to extremities and joints.

Asanas for the extremities

1. Utkatasana
2. Ek padasana
3. Gomukhasana

1.   Utkatasana—The Upraised Posture

When my body moves in a coordinated rhythm, synchronization and mindfulness increase.

The components of this asana's term translate to 'raised' (ut) and 'waist' (kati). As the name suggests, the aim of this asana is to raise your waist by rising on the heels, lowering the body and rising again.

Utkatasana enables great neuromuscular coordination. Awareness heightens and focus strengthens.

Method of Practice

Starting Position
1.   Stand erect, keep your hands at their respective sides and spread your legs by a foot's width. Focus your eyes at a point ahead.

Steps
1.   While inhaling, with palms facing down, raise both your hands parallel to each other, in front of the body up to shoulder-level.
2.   Simultaneously, raise your heels to stand on the toes.
3.   Exhaling, lower your body to a squatting position till your thighs press against the calves.
4.   Hold this squatting position, suspending your breath for 6 seconds.

Posture Release
1.   Inhaling, rise to your toes.

2. Take a pause on the toes, retaining your breath for 6 seconds.

3. Exhaling, lower your heels to the floor, bring the hands down and return to the starting position.

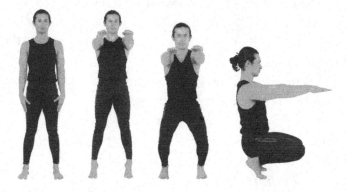

Limitations/Contraindications

- Moderate and severe arthritis of knees, acute deep vein thrombosis, sprained ankle, stiff joints, vertigo and sciatica pains.
- Do not suspend your breath if you are suffering from any cardiac condition.

Benefits

Physical

- Flexibility of your joints increases.
- The muscles of your legs and pelvis are strengthened.
- It enhances the balancing capacity of your body.
- It engages your core muscles.

Therapeutic
- With regular practice, you could lose weight, especially from your hips.
- It helps in relieving joint and back pains.

Psychological
- Regular practice improves balance and increases mental determination.
- It steadies the mind and sharpens focus.

Muscles Involved
- Quadriceps, gastrocnemius, soleus and intrinsic muscles of the foot
- Abductors and flexors of the shoulder
- Extensors of the legs, ankles and toes

My Variation for Utkatasana

Variation 1
1. Stand with your legs and heels together (you can adjust the distance of the heels slightly to maintain balance) and toes pointing outwards and sideways.
2. While inhaling, raise your hands to the shoulder-level from the front and simultaneously rise on your toes (but not too much).
3. Squat down so that your knees are spread wide apart as you exhale. Your hands remain extended at the shoulder-level.
4. Remain in this position for 6 seconds.
5. While inhaling, rise so that you are on your toes.

6.   Exhaling, lower your feet and hands.

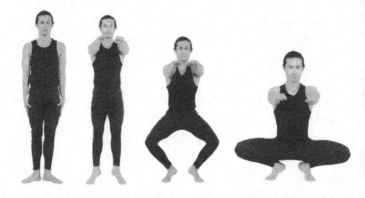

Variation 2

1.   There is no starting position.
2.   While keeping your body supported on your toes, raise your heels together, keep your knees wide apart and remain in the position as long as comfortable but not more than a minute.

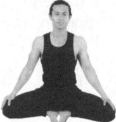

2.   Ekpadasana—The One Leg Posture

I resolve to remain equipoised as my goals are set high.

Achieving steadiness of body and mind is the primary aim of yoga. A steady body is a home to health, vitality and efficiency. Neuromuscular coordination and concentration of the mind enables this steadiness. There are yogic techniques with simple steps that harmonize the body and mind together. Ekpadasana is one such technique.

Method of Practice

Starting Position
1. Stand with your feet together and hands by your side.

Steps
1. Using your hands, lift your right leg laterally and press the sole of your foot against the left thigh as high as you can, the heel preferably close to the groin and toes pointing down. For those who cannot lift their legs so high, avoid placing the foot against your knees but rest the foot, wherever comfortable, against the thigh.
2. Balance your weight on the right leg.
3. Once balance is achieved, join both of your palms in a prayer pose. Breathe normally.
4. Maintain the pose for a few seconds. If your body sways or you tend to lose balance, try to fix your gaze at one point ahead.
5. Lower your leg and repeat the same procedure with the opposite leg
6. Gradually increase the timing of remaining in the posture from a few seconds to 1 minute with each leg.

Posture Release
1. Release your hands and lower your leg to stand with your feet together and hands on the sides.

Limitations/Contraindications
•   Severe arthritis, lower back pain, sciatica, slipped disc, or vertigo.

- Those with weak legs, lack of or very weak neuromuscular coordination may find it difficult to maintain the posture.

Benefits

Physical
- It strengthens the muscles of legs and spine.
- It improves your body balance, endurance and alertness.

Therapeutic
- Isometric contraction strengthens your muscle more efficiently as well as the bone it is attached to.
- It stimulates many areas of your nervous system.

Psychological
- It develops your sense of equilibrium.
- It sharpens your awareness and concentration.
- It keeps your mind in the present moment.
- It calms the mind.

Muscles Involved
- Flexors, abductors, external rotators of the hip and knee flexors of the hip that are bent.
- Flexors and extensors of the leg that are erect and gluteus muscles.

My Variation for Ekpadasana

Method of Practice
1. Lie on your back with your feet together and hands at the sides.

2. Keeping your left leg straight, bend the right knee laterally and place your heel near the groin or as high up as you can so that the entire heel of the right foot is placed firmly against the inner side of the left thigh.
3. Raise both your hands above the head to rest on the floor. Join your palms together.
4. Stay in this position for 6 seconds.
5. Release your hands and bring them to the sides and straighten your right leg.
6. Repeat with your left leg.

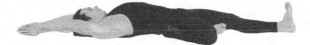

3. *Gaumukhasana—The Cow Head Posture*

When I am composed and calm, all actions flow effortlessly.

Gaumukhasana is conducive in order to establish harmony and rhythm which are most suited for concentration. It balances the two sides of the body, which is useful since we generally prefer either the left or the right side. It also stipulates a firm grounding.

Method of Practice

Starting Position
1. Sit with your legs fully outstretched.

Steps
1. Bend your left leg, bring it from under your right knee and place your heel near your right hip.

2. Bend your right leg, bring it over your left knee and place your heel near the left hip.
3. Raise your right hand straight up above your head and bend it at the elbow towards the back.
4. Take your other hand backwards from below, bend it at the elbow to grasp the right hand, interlocking your fingers as shown in the picture.
5. The head must remain straight and facing front.
6. Stay in this position as long as you are comfortable, however, not more than a minute is necessary.
7. Unclasp your fingers and return to the starting position.
8. Repeat with the opposite leg and hand.

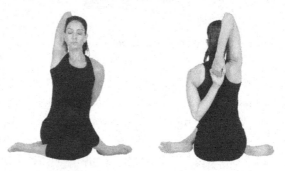

Limitations/Contraindications
- Severe arthritis of the shoulder joints or frozen shoulders
- Arthritis of the lower limbs

Benefits

Physical
- It improves blood flow to the pelvic region.

- It stretches the hips, thighs, ankles, chest, shoulders, arms and wrists.
- It loosens all your joints and stretches your spine.

Therapeutic
- It helps to relieve stiff shoulders.
- It helps to reduce backaches.
- It aids in treatment of sciatica.

Psychological
- Regular practice reduces stress.
- It develops calmness of mind.

Muscles Involved
- Wrist extensors.
- Shoulder rotator cuff.
- Forearms, thigh abductors and groin.

F. Asanas for relaxation

In today's fast-paced world, we seldom slow down to rest and relax. In fact, rest and relaxation have come to be somewhat negatively perceived in a world that values busyness and valourises hustle culture. Lack of rest causes unwanted stress and tension to the body and the mind. The number of people suffering from mental and emotional distress is increasing by the day. We are constantly doing things, forgetting to unwind and just be. Most of us find it difficult to meditate and relax because of the *rajasic* (restless) tendency of the mind that does not allow us to achieve mental quietude.

The aim of yoga is to introduce harmony and happiness to one's life. Asanas that enhance the passive awareness of our breathing help in relaxation of the body and the mind. They help to keep the mind at rest and the muscles free from tension. They also help one become aware and relax consciously. These benefits greatly help one to overcome fatigue, tension and stress.

Rest, relaxation and recovery are also crucial for maintaining health and vitality. Staying healthy doesn't just mean always being active, it also means learning when to slow down. Good health means striking a balance between movement and relaxation. Too much of either extreme can disturb mental and physical equanimity. Hence, practising relaxation asanas and passive breath awareness is equally critical to maintaining good physical and mental health.

Asanas for relaxation

1. Makarasana
2. Dhradasana
3. Shavasana

1. Makarasana—The Crocodile Posture

To just be is an achievement.

When one observes a crocodile, it appears as though it is constantly at rest unless stimulated. This pose is an effective technique for overcoming physical or mental fatigue and calming an agitated mind.

Method of Practice

Starting Position
1. Lie down on your stomach, head resting on your hands.
2. With your legs outstretched, keep your heels apart with your big toes touching each other.
3. Once in the position, remain motionless, letting go of all the weight on the ground.

Steps
1. Close your eyes and breathe normally and rhythmically.
2. Remain in this position for about 5 minutes.

Posture Release
1. Gently open your eyes.
2. Slowly turn to your right side for a few minutes before sitting up.

Limitations/Contraindications
- Psychological disorder—depression
- Cardiac conditions and pregnancy

Benefits

Physical
- There is deep relaxation for your shoulders and spine.
- It relaxes your body completely.

- It rejuvenates your entire body and mind.
- It helps to breathe slowly, efficiently and deeply.
- It relieves the mind and body tension.

Therapeutic
- It relieves muscular and nervous tension.
- There is relief from headaches, fatigue and insomnia.
- It reduces anxiety, calms the mind and releases tension.
- Conscious relaxation normalizes blood pressure, pulse rate and respiratory cycles.

Psychological
- It improves concentration and focus.
- It induces a meditative effect.
- It turns the mind inwards, calming it and preventing anxiety.

2.   Dhradhasana—The Firm Posture

To remain unaffected, being pure and peaceful is my aim.
     It is an effective technique to experience the rest of prolonged deep sleep in a short period.

Method of Practice

Starting Position
1.   Lie down with your legs stretched at full length, kept together in a relaxed manner.

Steps
1.   Gently turn and lie on the right side of the body.

2. Fold your right hand at the elbow and rest your head on the right forearm.
3. Your legs must be straight, the left leg over the right. In case you find keeping the legs straight difficult, you can bend the knees a little for balance.
4. Close your eyes and breathe normally. Avoid any movement of the body.
5. Maintain this relaxed breathing.
6. Gently turn and lie on the left side in the same manner.

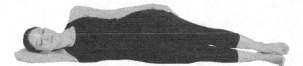

Variation
1. Lie on the side and bend the legs at the knee at a right angle. Follow the above method.

Posture Release
1. Gently open your eyes and sit up slowly with the support of your hands.

Limitations/Contraindications
Psychological disorders such as depression

Benefits

Physical
This posture favours ease of breathing.

Therapeutic
- It aids digestion.
- It relieves nocturnal emissions and stressful dreams.
- There is relief from headaches, fatigue and insomnia.
- Conscious relaxation normalizes the blood pressure, pulse rate and respiratory cycles.

Psychological
- It quickly rejuvenates the body and mind.
- It reduces anxiety, calms the mind and releases stress and tension.
- It induces a meditative effect.

3.   Shavasana—The Corpse Posture

I am at peace.

   True relaxation would mean a complete resignation of the body to the laws of gravity, the mind to nature. Whenever physical or mental fatigue is experienced or the mind is agitated, the practice of shavasana is recommended. The complete relaxation of the voluntary muscles at once transfers the energy to the involuntary parts. This transfer of energy by voluntary action and involuntary reaction produces the equilibrium necessary for the renewal of strength. Shavasana may either be partial shavasana or complete shavasana.

Partial Shavasana: Method of Practice

Starting Position
1.   Lie down on your back. Extend your arms by the sides such that they are not too far or too near the thighs. Keep your legs comfortably apart.

2. Once in this position, close your eyes and remain motionless throughout the practice.

Steps
1. Breathe rhythmically, subtly and slowly.
2. Avoid any movement of the body mentally relax the sixteen vital zones (Marmasthanan) of the body, by paying attention to each part separately, i.e., your toes, knees, thighs, hands, arms, groin, pelvis, navel, abdomen, chest, neck, lips, tip of the nose, eyes, space between the eyebrows, forehead and the crown of the head.
3. Maintain this relaxed state for about 10–15 minutes.

Posture Release
1. Gently open your eyes and lie on the right side for a few minutes before sitting up.

Complete Shavasana

Starting Position
1. Same as above.

Steps
1. Close your eyes and follow the normal rhythmic breathing.
2. Avoiding any movement of the body, consciously switch off all nervous stimuli.
3. Maintain this state for about 15–20 minutes.

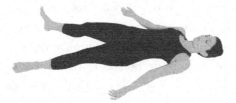

Posture Release
1. Gently open your eyes and lie on the right side for a few minutes before sitting up.

Limitations / Contraindications
Psychological disorders such as depression.

Benefits

Physical
•   It relieves muscular and nervous tension.
•   It stimulates blood circulation.

Therapeutic
•   There is relief from headaches, fatigue and insomnia.
•   It reduces anxiety, calms the mind and releases stress and tension.
•   Conscious relaxation normalizes blood pressure, pulse rate and respiratory cycles.

Psychological
•   It improves concentration and focus.
•   It has mentally restorative benefits and invigorates the entire body.
•   It induces a meditative effect.

Now let's add a power booster to your asana practice: Yogendra Rhythm. In order to maximize the results of your asana practice, it is important to correlate the movements of the body with a specific breathing rhythm. Breath plays a crucial, indispensable role in yoga. Without an awareness of your breath, you are not practising asanas, merely stretching your body mindlessly and mechanically. Awareness is of utmost importance while practising asanas, otherwise, you may succumb to unwanted injury and pain or be caught in your mental loop of thoughts and worry. Rhythmic breathing can help us become aware of our body's movements.

Shri Yogendraji developed a special breathing rhythm for asana practice. This systematic and scientific practice is known as the Yogendra rhythm. In a Yogendra rhythm, our inhalation and exhalation patterns coordinate with the contraction and expansion of the chest and abdomen. Here's how it goes: breathe in, expanding your chest and abdomen for two counts. Next, hold your breath for double the length of your inhalation for four counts. Exhale, contracting your chest and abdomen for two counts. Hold your empty lungs for four counts. When the lungs are full, we call the waiting period 'holding' or 'retention' as we are holding the breath or retaining the air inside our lungs. When lungs are empty, we call this period 'suspension' as we are suspending breathing. Retention and suspension of breath serve two main purposes. Firstly, doing so purifies the blood fully and flushes toxins from the body more effectively. Secondly, it gives the mind a pause to absorb and become more aware.

Shri Yogendraji, after a lot of experiential practice and research, arrived at a balanced ratio of breathing. He observed that a breathing ratio of 1:2:1 is the most beneficial. This means that the retention or suspension of breath is twice the amount of inhalation or exhalation. For example, the breathing rhythm of 2:4:2 indicates 2 seconds of inhalation, 4 seconds of retention and 2 seconds of exhalation. You can increase the ratio to 3:6:3 or 4:8:4, depending upon your practice and capacity. However, the ratio of 1:2:1 should always be observed. The Yogendra rhythm of breathing should always be followed while practising asanas.

There are various benefits to incorporating the Yogendra rhythm in your asana practice. It makes your practice easier and more comfortable. It increases lung capacity, improves breathing and makes the practice of pranayama easier. Most importantly, it increases awareness and mindfulness while practising asanas, making the practice of asanas beneficial for overall health and providing physical and holistic benefits to the body. Moreover, retention of breath provides better oxygenation of blood while suspension helps flush toxins from the body through the medium of breath. Coordinating bodily movements with your breath helps reduce physical tension and fatigue, making you feel active and energetic after your asana practice instead of tired and sore.

Now let's take a quick look at some dos and don'ts for your asana practice:
Allocate a time for regular practice. Thirty to 40 minutes of uninterrupted daily practice is suggested. This duration can be gradually increased to one hour.

The best time for asana practice is in the morning before breakfast or any other suitable time on an empty stomach, with a minimum gap of three to four hours after the last meal you have consumed. Never practice asanas on a full stomach. The only asana that can be done immediately after a meal is *vajrasana* as it promotes digestion

Begin every asana with a conditioning of the mind. Set aside 5-10 minutes to help bring the mind to a place of calm and quietude before you begin the practice.

After conditioning, warm up properly by practising sahajbhavasanas and then proceed to practising asanas.

Ideally, begin with standing asanas, followed by seated asanas, followed by asanas on your abdomen and lastly, asanas on the back. End each session with a few minutes of shavasana to seal the practice and relax the body and mind completely.

Do not skip the conditioning exercises of sahajbhavasanas or shavasana when carrying out your practice.

Wear breathable and comfortable clothes during your yoga practice, not tight and uncomfortable clothing which restrict the movement of the body and the breath.

Choose a well-ventilated room.

Ensure that there is minimal distraction during the time allotted to your asana practice. Avoid practising directly under the fan or setting your air-conditioning at low temperatures. It is ideal to practice in a place which has a natural flow of breeze. If that is not feasible, avoid extreme temperatures in the room selected for your practice.

Use a personal yoga mat for your practice. Choose a yoga mat that is made from natural fibres, anti-skid and easily washable. Hygiene and comfort are equally important for your asana practice. Avoid sharing yoga mats and invest in one of your own.

Asana practice should be done with absolute concentration and awareness of breath. There should be a conscious effort towards reaching the final posture without rushing or torturing the body to achieve it. Steadiness of posture combined with ease is more important than reaching the final posture.

The practice of asanas must be graceful, rhythmic and mindful. The breath should be synchronized with all movements, in accordance with Yogendra rhythm. Lack of awareness of breath makes your practice mechanical and mindless. Being focused and aware will give you holistic benefits of the practice more than merely going through an asana practice session mechanically and fast.

Do not overdo any asana, especially if you are a beginner. Give your body and mind time to adjust to the practice and gradually and gracefully progress with your practice.

As far as possible, practice under the guidance and advice of a trained yoga teacher. This will help you avoid unwanted injury and pain and also help rectify incorrect alignment and posture.

Now the question on everyone's mind, 'What exactly is the benefit I will get from a regular asana practice?' It's not wrong to want to know about the eventual result; however, don't also focus overly on the final goal at the expense of everything else. Here are the tangible benefits that should arise as a result of regular asana practice:

A strong and supple body, greater endurance level, a tool to help reduce excess weight or maintain a healthy weight.

A strong and flexible spine with enhanced spinal circulation.

Healthy and strong digestive organs and abdominal muscles, since the practice of asanas focuses on the compression and stretching of the abdominal region.

A healthy and disease-free mind and body. You will notice an improvement in concentration and enhanced awareness and mindfulness.

Regular practice of asanas helps prevent as well as cure diseases and can be used as a complementary and alternative healing therapy.

Improved flexibility and less stiffness and tension in the body.

Asana practice is an alternative remedy for bodily aches. Regular practice effectively reduces pain in the joints, muscles, spine and extremities

Improved blood circulation in the body, which in turn helps to keep the internal organs healthy.

Helps one feel energetic and active after the practice.

Induces a sense of calmness and quietude in the mind, if practised correctly with mindful movements of the body with the breath.

As special take-away for my readers, here's a curated list of asanas if you are looking for some that will help you deal with a particular issue or if you just want to rejuvenate after a long day at work.

Instant Rejuvenation

This set of asanas can be your go-to remedies whenever you need to feel instantly refreshed. Give them a go!
- Bhujangasan
- Shalabhasan
- Ushtrasan
- Makarasan

Calming
Are you constantly stressed or anxious? Don't be. Life is too short to worry. But if you still can't help being worrywart, we've got you covered with these asanas:
- Badrasana
- Yogamudra
- Dridasana
- Shavasana

Digestive

Feeling a little under the weather with your tummy? Or do you routinely overstuff your digestive tract, making it work overtime all year? We may have something that might help.

- Vajrasan
- Ardhamatsyaendrasan
- Sitting Vajrasan
- Pavanmuktasan

Office (Sitting Asanas)

Yes, that's right! We have some asanas that you can do right at your office desk as well. They are easy and simple but can help you immensely with your flexibility and relieve you of all those aches and pains that you typically feel after a long session of work.

Do the following flow in office:

- Neck exercises
- Wrist and hand exercises
- Cat and cow pose
- Tratak

Relaxing flow

- Badrasana
- Pavanmuktasana
- Lying down vakrasana
- Nispand Bhav Meditation
- Pranayama no. 4

Afterword

From Stressors to Joysters

RESET is a very powerful word. When you decide to reset, you can go from struggling professionally to being a competent and valuable professional asset to any organisation. Once you decide to reset, you can pivot from a series of unsatisfying and draining relationships to expressing your truest self in a real, meaningful and deep relationship. When you decide to RESET, you can shift from into a state of financial abundance and material prosperity. But for all this more you need to make the decision to Reset. You need to be willing to put in the work to Reset. And if you are ready to that then this book will help you in every possible way. Many a times I meet people who are extremely successful professionally, but their personal life is a veritable mess. Other times people have a lot of love and happiness in their relations, but financial stress work-worries do not let them enjoy what they have. And in yet another scenario if things are working well at the home and work fronts then your body is in a mess with blood-pressure, diabetes, cholesterol and other lifestyle diseases.

It always disturbed me immensely that our life, though so full of material prosperity was rife with challenges on so many fronts. It was as if we had to wait for this to go wrong or that to go wrong; only then would life seem real. That shouldn't be so. With that idea in mind, I wrote *Seven Rules to Reset Your Mind and Body for Greater Well-Being*, so that you could have one go-to for any and every problem or challenge that life may throw your way. The seven aspects that this book looks at were chosen to help you address the major causes of stress and anxiety in modern life. With *Seven Rules . . .* in your hands these will turn from stressors to *joysters* of your life.

See, we may want many things in life; most of our unhappiness and dissatisfaction comes from not having what we think we should have. But try working with the tips and tricks in these five chapters and you will be on the way to having what you need most to reset your life. These chapters are filled with the life-experiences of real people and the Yoga Institute's rich legacy of knowledge in creating practical, relatable solutions for the real problems of real people. And if you are a little lost with all that you have read then I have quick Reset re-look for you right here.

Resetting our work-life becomes non-negotiable when we hear of 20–30-year-olds dying from heart attacks or suffering from grave lifestyle diseases. Needless to say, these deeply disturbing occurrences are caused by the increasingly stress prone nature of our jobs and careers. It is a fact that there is no escape from work but that does not mean we that we lose our lives for the work we do. Or for that matter even compromise our health and family-life in the name of work and career. I like an analogy I read somewhere that was shared by an American politician. When we keep working mindlessly it drains our life's energy in the longer run. Use Reset your Work-Life when you find that you are working mindlessly for the sake of working. Use Reset when you find that you are working in a hurry or you are working to fulfil needs that you have simply created. Use this chapter when you find yourself comparing your life to others. Remember if work is giving you aches and pains or sleepless nights or wreaking havoc on your personal life then it is time to reset!

Resetting your Perception leads you into the possibilities of your life that you withhold from yourself through negativity and limiting attitudes. Our mind has a tendency to attach undue value to unpleasant events and provoke extreme decisions and behaviors. But remember life is too short to be angry and unhappy, even temporarily, let alone for longer periods of time. We have become anxiety-driven and survival-obsessed. We are habituated to constantly being critical, dissatisfied and blind to all that is good in things, situations, and people. That is where resetting your perception will help you. From being survival driven you will become more acceptance-driven. You will shift from Finding faults to finding value even in the mundane and the ordinary. Once you train your mind to see the good, once you train to reset your perception you will find that joy and ease flow into your life. But this needs both time and effort. If you are ready to put in the work Reset your Perception will give you all the tools you need to re-work your thought patterns and mind blocks and reset for life.

With Reset your Social Life we look at the increasing distances and social isolation that has crept into all our lives.

In our grand plans for success, we often assume that people are unimportant and unnecessary. But in doing that we forget that a single stick is only as strong as one stick. But when that stick is in a bundle of sticks it becomes as strong the entire bundle.

Our social interactions and social networks do much more than help us know one and other. For one, they act as an emotional support system. Next, they are excellent at helping us de-stress. Just think how much fun you used to have as kids after a game or two with your friends. Didn't you feel light and happy? And why do you think you feel so heavy and fatigued all the time now? It is because of the absence of a balanced and vibrant social life. Remember it's not about how big your social circle is, it is about how genuine it is. Reset your Social-Life will address the common mistakes we all make while forming social connections. It will also look at grave missteps and suggest viable detours for you. Remember the greatest things that happen to our lives are hidden in the smallest moments of human connection. Missing out on human connection and bonding is missing out on life itself.

Reset your Relationship is as it sounds: it addresses the proverbial black sheep that relationships have become for all of us. Reset your Relationship intends to remind us what relationships are really about. It is, has been and will always be about love and care. This chapter will try to remove the extra layers, the complications, the unnecessary flab as it were that has crept into our relationships. Nine out of ten times relationships become difficult when we are scared: scared of the change the relationship will bring into our life or scared of being rejected when they see us as we are without filters. Reset your Relationship is about learning to not ignore the best in life by fearing the best in life. A relationship reset will mentor you in accepting yourself first. Because without love for the self how can there be love for another? Look at relationships from a place of stability, comfort and growth and that is how you begin the journey of this emotional reset.

Any reset of our life is impossible if we do not look at sleep, food and exercise. These are the three most underestimated power-factors in our life. For instance, if we are unwell our food has the capacity to become medicine, to heal us. Someone very truly said once that we are what we eat. So, if you look at the layers of flab on your body you will see the result of whatever you ate. Your body is literally made of what you put into it. Similarly, exercise has the potential to do wonders for our body not only physically but also emotionally and mentally. Just ask yourself what can you do without the support of a healthy body. Yet we do not spend time caring for our bodies glued as we are to our gadgets. As we spend hours bent over our gadgets, our spines curve, our muscles become loose, our arteries get choked and we put heaps and heaps of visceral fat on all our organs. And finally sleep. Just ask about the importance of sleep to a woman or man who has not had a good night's sleep. Without sleep you won't have the energy to get through the day leave alone getting to your goals. Any doubt about the importance of sleep as a biological function that is at the core of mental and physical well-being is ill-founded and misplaced. Sleep is vital to our lives as humans. So, if your parents scolded you as child for sleeping too much now it's time to read the book and tell them about the wonders of good sleep.

So, there you have it, I have put my years of learning and hours of long yet loving labour into the writing of this book. This has been a labour of love for me and I hope that it will serve you well. I have crafted the seven dimensions of the book with the firm belief that if we address these seven aspects of our lives, we are well on our way to living a healthy, balanced and joyful life. That is my gift to you in this book.

Enjoy.

Namaskar.